CHARLES VAN RIPER, editor *Foundations of Speech Pathology Series*

Prentice-Hall Foundations of Speech Pathology Series

PRENTICE-HALL INTERNATIONAL, INC., *London*
PRENTICE-HALL OF AUSTRALIA, PTY., LTD., *Sydney*
PRENTICE-HALL OF CANADA, LTD., *Toronto*
PRENTICE-HALL OF INDIA (PRIVATE) LTD., *New Delhi*
PRENTICE-HALL OF JAPAN, INC., *Tokyo*
PRENTICE-HALL DE MEXICO, S.A., *Mexico City*

Delayed Speech
and
Language Development

Delayed Speech
and
Language Development

NANCY E. WOOD

Research Director
The John Tracy Clinic
Los Angeles

Prentice-Hall, Inc., *Englewood Cliffs, N. J.*

For Orne E. Wood

My teacher, counselor, companion, friend—
and not so incidentally—my mother

editor's note

THE SET OF VOLUMES WHICH CONSTITUTES THE *Foundations of Speech Pathology Series* is designed to serve as the nucleus of a professional library, both for students of speech pathology and audiology and for the practicing clinician. Each individual text in the series is written by an author whose authority has long been recognized in his field. Each author has done his utmost to provide the basic information concerning the speech or hearing disorders covered in his book. Our new profession needs new tools, good ones, to be used not once but many times. The flood of new information already upon us requires organization if it is to be assimilated and if it is to help us solve the many different professional problems which beset us. This series provides that essential organization.

One of the unifying and outstanding features of all the volumes in this series is the use of search items. In addition to providing the core of information concerning his subject, each author has indicated clearly other sources having significance for the topic being discussed. The reader is urged to explore, to search, and to discover—and the trails are charted. In so rapidly changing a profession as ours, we cannot afford to remain content with what we have been taught. We must learn to continue learning.

Although each individual volume in this series is complete unto itself, the instructor should welcome the opportunity presented by the *Foundations of Speech Pathology Series* to combine several volumes to form the basic structure of the course he teaches. They may also be used as collateral readings. These short but comprehensive books give the instructor a thoroughly flexible teaching tool. But the primary aim of the authors of these texts has been the creation of a basic library for all of our students and professional workers. In this series we have sought to provide a common fund of knowledge to help unify and serve our new profession.   ❧❧❧   *ix*

before we begin

NEARLY EVERY NONFICTION BOOK WRITTEN THESE DAYS CONTAINS a preface, a prologue, a foreword, or some special section where the author explains the purpose of the book, describes how or why it happened to be written, and acknowledges those "many people" who were instrumental in helping to get the final copy into print.

It is difficult to decide if such a section is appropriate here, for if all the people who were involved in the preparation of this small volume were listed, name by name, the acknowledgments would be longer than the text. And, if it seemed appropriate to describe why and how this book was written, it would be necessary to state that it was not written *because* of anything. It was, however, written *in spite* of a number of things. It was written in spite of the fact that it addresses itself to a subject which is much too encompassing to be covered thoroughly by any book, regardless of size. It was written in spite of the fact that its intent is not so much to provide answers to questions as it is to raise a few. It was written also in spite of the fact that, with such a wealth of available material about delayed speech and language development written under various titles and from numerous vantage points, an all-inclusive organization of this information remains improbable, if not impossible.

If truth is required, this book was written for selfish reasons entirely. It provided the writer with an opportunity to tell students who had decided to major in the field of communication disorders that they had selected one of the most provocative, challenging, and constantly stimulating areas of study available. It gave the writer a chance to applaud those university professors concerned with the professional preparation of Speech Pathologists and Audiologists for their demanding, rigorous, dedicated commitment to excellence. It supplied an occasion to commend those clinicians and researchers who have assumed the awesome responsibility of providing and improving diagnostic and therapeutic services for children with communication disorders, recognizing that these endeavors require sober reflection and constant exploration.

There may not be a single new idea recorded here, for what has been written was gleaned from numerous conversations with directors of clinics, supervisors, classroom teachers, researchers, clinicians, professors, therapists, and specialists from various disciples throughout the country. Some points of view reflect the feelings of parents of children with delayed speech and language development which they expressed in many searching and complex discussions. The most salient facts, perhaps, resulted from working with and observing the children themselves, the majority of whom did not say a word.

This book does not purport to answer all questions about delayed speech and language development. It lays no claim to unique ideas or revolutionary theories. If, by chance, it might in some way stimulate a new thought, or provoke a fresh idea, or communicate the need for further study, it will have more than served its purpose.

N.E.W.

contents

chapter III

chapter IV

DELAYED SPEECH AND LANGUAGE DEVELOPMENT OCCURS WITH GREATER frequency and, at times, with greater complexity than any other known communication disorder. Consequently, the evaluation of delayed speech and language development demands unstinting rigor and considerable clinical competence if the various possible causal factors of this problem are to be differentiated. To some degree, both the frequency and the complexity of delayed speech and language development seem to have increased during the last decade. This apparent increase is due, at least partially, to several factors.

First, in this supersonic age in which we live, with its television, telephone, and telespatial communications, there is a tendency for adults to impose stricter demands on young children for earlier

1 speech and language development

and more accurate speech development than ever before. Parents, teachers, siblings, relatives—even neighbors seemingly join in a concerted effort to remind children of the need to speak effectively and clearly. During the last two or three decades, our levels of aspiration for speech development and other areas of learned behavior, like the cost of living, have gone up. In fact, in some families, effective speech has become a sort of status symbol. Therefore, when contrasted with children of the 1940's or the 1950's, children today must learn to communicate very early and on a much more complex level—often because of an emphasis placed upon the need for effective speech as a social tool.

1 For an interesting exploration of the fascination of language, including latest discoveries and research in communication, read Language: A Modern Synthesis, written by Joshua Whatmough. Available in a paperback edition from Mentor Books, The New American Library of World Literature, Inc., 501 Madison Avenue, New York 22, N. Y. Chapter X, "Language: Society, Individual and Symbol," is particularly pertinent to this discussion.

Second, more parents have become aware of developmental schedules and the many factors that may interrupt normal development.

Through such popular professional writings as those by Spock, Gesell, Ilg, and Ames, parents are more aware of what a child should be doing at various stages of normal development. With this more critical awareness, parents are seeking professional help more quickly and earlier than they have in the past. They want to know if their child is significantly delayed in speech and language development, and, if so, what can be done to alleviate or to solve the problem.

2   Further discussion of this point can be found in Dorothea McCarthy's article, "Language Disorders and Parent-Child Relationships," which appeared in the Journal of Speech and Hearing Disorders, XIX: 4 (December 1954), 514-23.

Third, medical science has made significant advances in reducing the mortality rate at birth. Today, more children are living who previously would have expired at birth. At the same time, many of the children who have survived traumatic deliveries are found later in life to have subtle and sometimes confusing disorders. Frequently, one of these disorders is a reduced capacity to communicate verbally, for many of these children do not learn to talk at the expected time or with the expected accuracy.

3   A thorough discussion of various disorders occurring in childhood is available in Clinical Management of Behavior Disorders in Children, written by two pediatricians, Harry Bakwin and Ruth Bakwin (Philadelphia and London: W. B. Saunders Co., 1960).

Finally, the development of new tests, the availability of new clinical services, the wealth of new information from research and the promise of more to come, have all sharpened the abilities of specialists to detect the presence of speech and language problems at an earlier age. Even more important, our knowledge of what to do about these various problems after they have been detected has shown rapid strides during the last decade. Fortunately, we are now less content to use the term *delayed speech* as an isolated classification of speech problem, and there seems to be fairly universal recognition that, because speech can be delayed by many factors, the treatment and education of children with delayed speech development must be related to the cause or causes of the delay.

4 Margaret H. Powers describes some of the problems connected with the use of the term *delayed speech* in her chapter on "Functional Disorders of Articulation-Symptomatology and Etiology," in L. E. Travis, ed., *Handbook of Speech Pathology* (New York: Appleton-Century-Crofts, Inc., 1957), pp. 707-68.

For these and other reasons, more and more children—particularly those between the ages of two and five—are being referred to clinics, diagnostic centers, or specialists in private practice because they do not communicate adequately. Concomitantly, there also has been an increase in the number of children who, when they reach school age, cannot participate effectively in routine classroom activities because of severely delayed speech and language development.

When these children are seen for initial examination in clinical settings throughout the country, there is a familiar ring to the statements made by each set of parents as they begin to discuss their child's problem: "Billy doesn't seem to be developing speech as he should. He doesn't pay attention to me when I talk to him. He doesn't seem to understand what I am saying." Or, "The other children in the neighborhood make fun of the way my child talks. Every day he runs home crying because the other children have teased him about his speech. He is becoming very difficult to manage." Or, "My younger child is beginning to imitate the 'baby talk' of my older child. I try to teach them both the correct way to say words, but it doesn't help." Or, "Jack seems to understand everything I say to him, but he still won't talk. He seems to be withdrawing into a world of his own. His younger sister isn't like that; she talks very well." Or, "I know my child is retarded, but if he could talk, I know we could teach him other things."

And, as the evaluations continue, there is also another familiar theme in the questions parents ask: "How important is speech and language development? What is delayed speech? When is speech considered delayed? What causes delayed speech? Should I be concerned if my child is not talking at two years of age? Does delayed speech run in families? How should I manage this problem at home? How frequently does this problem occur? What can be done about it?" Questions such as these form a basis for what often becomes a complicated, time-consuming, intricate, and multiphasic clinical study. Our task here is to obtain answers for these and similar questions by exploring normal communication processes and by considering the causal factors, methods of evaluation, and some possible therapeutic or educational approaches to delayed speech and language development. To do this, we must be convinced of the importance of speech and language development to total growth and maturation.

THE IMPORTANCE OF SPEECH AND LANGUAGE DEVELOPMENT

To say that speech and language development is an important aspect of human growth is to express neither a new concept nor a debatable one. Man's need to communicate effectively through speech has been emphasized throughout the ages by those who have helped shape the destiny of our world. Philosophers, politicians, statesmen, dictators, judges, teachers, ministers—all these and many more—have recognized and cherished the value of the spoken word, well spoken. To say, then, that speech and language development is important is like saying that the education of man is important, or that the communication of ideas is important, or—in a civilized society—that man's ability to relate to man is important. Of course, it is important; but the question is: to whom is it important, and why?

Specialists in speech and hearing disorders have as their primary professional responsibility the study of the normal speech and hearing processes and the many factors that may hinder or impede oral communication. Realistically, however, this responsibility is shared with specialists from various disciplines, for speech and language development is a multidiscipline concern. Scientists and educators involved with learning, both as a process and an end product, are intensely aware of the importance of speech development as it pertains to learning. Because of this awareness, they regard that period of time when a child first uses speech to communicate as a critical stage in his total growth pattern. Actually, the onset of speech marks that time when a child first becomes an individual, separate from his mother, for it is through the use of speech for communication that a child first has ideas of his own and a new way to express them.

Educators emphasize the importance of speech development and the refinement of the speech process, for they recognize that successful learning situations, both within and outside the classroom, depend upon a child's ability to understand and use words.

Physicians have recognized the importance of speech and language development for many years, and they attempt to obtain information about a child's speech development, realizing that such information provides major clues for predicting a child's total developmental schedule. For this reason, when a physician examines a young child, speech development is usually one area of major concern to him, and during the examination, he may ask many questions about the way in which the child communicates at home. How does he tell you what he wants? How does he make his wants known? How many words can he use now? These are the routine questions that physicians ask the mothers of young children.

5 Physicians frequently consider the problem of delayed speech and language development from different viewpoints, according to their particular professional interest. Compare the comments made by J. T. Morrow in "A Psychiatrist Looks at the Non-Verbal Child," *Exceptional Child,* XXV (1959), 347-51, with those discussed by I. Rapin in "The Neurologist Looks at the Non-Verbal Child," *Exceptional Children,* XXVI (1959), 48-52.

Psychologists, too, have both an academic interest in the development of speech and a professional concern for the many factors that can hinder or impede its use. One of the reasons psychologists are interested in speech development is that psychological tests, particularly those designed to assess the intelligence or intellectual potential of young children, require communication between examiner and child. Although performance tests provide a possible avenue through which a child's mental abilities can be explored without using speech, it is well known that verbal scales, such as vocabulary tests, and general information questions provide much more accurate information about the level of intelligence than any other single type of test criterion. For this reason, psychologists must have considerable knowledge about the development of speech and language and the ways in which speech development can be delayed. They must also be aware of the many causes of delayed speech and the effects of this delay on the child, his parents, and others in his environment.

6 See Melvin E. Allerhand, "Psychological Assessment of the Non-Verbal Child," in N. Wood *Monographs of the Society for Research in Child Development,* XXV:3 (1963), 49-57.

Counselors in vocational guidance and career selection also recognize the importance of developing good speech patterns, for they know that automation and other forms of vocational streamlining are almost certain to eliminate numerous jobs that currently do not require complicated verbal exchanges. Because today's child seems predestined to live in a world that will place high priorities on the spoken word, it is logical to conclude that in future years there will be a greater need for abstract thinking "on the job," and that communication through speech will be an even more complex process.

These, of course, are just a few of the specialists in the medical, paramedical, scientific, educational, and habilitative fields who have stressed the importance of speech and language development. Certainly, sociologists, linguists, anthropologists, special education teachers, physical therapists, and occupational therapists contribute greatly to the better understanding of normal communication processes and of the many factors that may interrupt this development.

The purpose here is not to attempt to discuss all of the areas of specialization which might relate in some way to the study of speech and language development, but rather to emphasize that speech and language development is a multiphasic process and that the study of delayed speech and language development requires a multidiscipline approach.

DEFINITION OF LANGUAGE

Most people know, at least vaguely, what *language* is. Yet, the term *language* is frequently interchanged with the term *speech* Actually, *language* is the broader, more encompassing term, referring to a learned process of which *speech* is one part. By definition, language is an organized system of linguistic symbols (words) ,

7   For a clear picture of speech as a part of language the volume *Foreign Accent* by Fred Chreist, in the Foundations of Speech Pathology Series (Englewood Cliffs, N. J.: Prentice-Hall, Inc., 1964), will be most helpful. Also, see John Carroll's *The Study of Language: A Survey of Linguistics and Related Disciplines in America* (Cambridge: Harvard University Press, 1953).

used by human beings to communicate on an abstract level. Language, then, is basic to all communication through words, encompassing reading and writing as well as the spoken word. It is, therefore, through language that we express our feelings, discuss our ideas, and present our points of view. It is through language that we share our experiences with others, describing for them our impressions or memories of people we have met, places we have been, or things we have seen. It is also through language that we can speak or write about an object without the necessity of having the object present; or, if we wish, we can through language discuss an abstract idea with which we have had no personal experience. Not only can we recall the past and discuss the present, but by means of language we can engage in the height of abstraction—we can discuss what may happen in the future. Language, then, has a predictive value.

8   In the two books, *The Art of Thinking,* by Ernest Dimnet (New York: Fawcett World Library, 1961), and *Words and Things,* by Roger Brown (Glencoe, Ill.: Free Press, 1958), language and language development is discussed in a lively and interesting manner. Both books should add measurably to the understanding of the magic and miracle of language and of its development.

Because of the great flexibility of language, communication with others stimulates our thinking, enlarges our symbol system, and helps organize our ideas. In a sense, communication begets communication, and, as the language experiences of an individual increase, so does his ability to operate symbolically on a more complex and abstract level. It should be clear, therefore, that the process of linguistic growth does not terminate with childhood, even though the development of language makes its greatest strides during that period of life.

The intricate process of language development is dependent upon the organism's abilities to receive, integrate, and express linguistic symbols. These linguistic symbols are received through two of the major sensory channels: vision and audition. Reception of the *written* word is achieved through reading; reception of the *spoken* word, through listening. As a correlate, the expression of language finds its outlet through *writing* and *speaking*. These functions, of course, require vision, audition, and motor skills. In addition, both the reception of language and its expression can be modified by the many cumulative functions of man, such as intelligence, perception, motivation, and other factors which increase the complexity of the language process.

9   For an analysis of the way in which language is learned, see O. H. Mowrer, "Hearing and Speaking: An Analysis of Language Learning," *Journal of Speech Disorders*, XXIII (1958), 143-52. According to Mowrer, what role does imitation play in language learning?

Even more complex than either the reception or the expression of language is the way in which the individual *integrates* linguistic symbols. This integration entails numerous aspects of thought behavior, such as: memory, recall, cognition, imagery, and association. Briefly, language is an organized set of symbols used for communication; an interrelation—actually, a union—of the reception, integration, and expression of information. In order to develop a language system, the organism must be able to receive stimuli and classify them by coding, sorting, selecting, organizing, and retaining this incoming information. Then, these informational bits can be translated into a verbal context prior to reading, writing, or speaking.

DEFINITION OF SPEECH

In brief, *speech* is the oral expression of language, beginning with the birth cry and continuing through many stages of development before it becomes a useful communication tool. Serious students of speech and language development never cease to be amazed that man has no anatomical or physiological structure used solely for the purpose of speech. For example, in order to speak, we use parts of our bodies intended to serve more basic functions. The lungs, designed to maintain life by providing the body with oxygen, also provide the air necessary for speech. The glottis, originally intended as a passage which can supply the body with food, is also used for phonation. The teeth and tongue, used initially for chewing food and forcing it down the gullet, are also the articulators of speech sounds.

Another thought-provoking fact is that, of all the language skills, speech is the only medium of expression that is not taught routinely by a special curriculum. Both reading and writing are regarded as skills which need special methods and procedures before a child can be expected to learn them. Yet, when speech is broken down into separate developmental stages, there is a tendency to consider this a simple process, and it may appear that a child passes effortlessly and surely from one stage to another. Perhaps this is the reason we tend to take speech development for granted, and that often it is only when something interrupts or delays this development that we question why such a delay has occurred.

Speech is a learned process—we are not born with either the desire or the need to speak. We learn to speak only because those around us use this method of communication; if we had been born to a culture where sounds or vocal noises were sufficient for communication, we would not have developed verbal language.

Like all types of learned behavior, speech development depends upon the maturation of the individual. Maturation determines *when* behavior can be learned, for maturation establishes certain periods of life when the organism has established a so-called "readiness" to learn a given activity.

> 10 The recognition of this "readiness" is a major factor in the success of a speech and hearing specialist to obtain maximum results with children who are delayed in speech and language development. More about speech readiness can be found in Clarence T. Simon's chapter, "The Development of Speech," in L. E. Travis, ed., *Handbook of Speech Pathology* (New York: Appleton-Century-Crofts, Inc., (1957), pp. 3-43.

Speech sounds develop in a series of stages that proceed from *prelinguistic* utterances through the linguistic use of symbols. The prelinguistic stage of development begins with nonmeaningful reflexive sounds which are related to the physiological changes in the infant during the first three months of life. From the third to the sixth month, the child gives evidence of responding to his own verbal play. It has been rather clearly proved that babies do not develop speech sounds during this period of nonpurposeful vocalization by imitating adults, but rather by imitating their own babblings. Hence, babbling is not true speech; it has no symbolic value. Rather, it is an autostimulation process whereby the child produces sounds randomly and then responds to his own vocalizations.

Developmentally, between the sixth and ninth months, a refinement period occurs, and toward the end of this stage the child begins to produce paired syllables (for example: *bye-bye; mama; dada; bebe*). These repetitive sounds are classified too often by anxious parents as speech. Actually, these repetitive sounds are

11   This is what Jean Piaget refers to as the egocentric period of language
      development in his book, The Origins of Intelligence in Children (New
      York: International Universities Press, Inc., 1952). When and why does
      the child turn from the egocentric to the social use of sound?

not true speech, for they have no symbolic value. However, repetitions such as these form the basic groundwork for the development of speech.

Up to this point, the average child's speech development can be predicted with a fair degree of accuracy, without too much concern for differences in environment. It is at this stage (6 to 9 months), however, and in the months that follow, that some children are found to proceed more rapidly in speech development than do others. Although there are many influences which seemingly play a part in this development, environmental differences are of major importance, and it has been demonstrated that a verbally rich environment can accelerate the child's rate of speech development.

12   The babbling stage of speech development is reviewed in H. R. Mykle-
      bust's article, "Babbling and Echolalia in Language Theory," Journal
      of Speech and Hearing Disorders, XXII (September 1957), No. 3, 356-60.
      Why is babbling so important to normal language development?

From 18 months to two years, a child usually acquires between 10 and 20 words which he can use meaningfully. Most of these words are nouns, usually the names of people or things. This is the period of *echoic* speech. During this time, children may imitate words used by adults perfectly, even to intonation and inflection, without knowledge of what the words mean. This is also the period when a child may string various sounds together or develop words that may have meaning for him but for no one else. This type of controlled vocalization is commonly referred to as *jargon*.

13   Compare the description of jargon in Charles Van Riper, Teaching Your
      Child to Talk (New York: Harper & Row, Publishers, 1950) with that in
      M. M. Lewis, Infant Speech: A Study of the Beginning of Language,
      2nd Ed. (London: Routledge & Kegan Paul, Ltd., 1951).

Twins have been known to develop the use of jargon to such a level of perfection that they can communicate easily with one another, and to the total exclusion of anyone else. This unique communication system has been termed *idioglossia*. Jargon normally decreases rapidly during this phase, so that by the time the child is approaching his second birthday, his use of jargon is negligible.

Between the second and third years, a greater growth in vocabulary occurs, within a shorter period of time, than in any other period of life. Part of this growth in vocabulary is due to the fact that sometime during this period children discover the use of "the question." As any adult who has spent time in the company of a three-year-old can testify, questioning becomes a major communication tool for youngsters of this age. From this point on, the child's speech and language development becomes a process of refinement and growth. Vocabulary increases and sentence structure becomes more complex. As a social being, the child depends more and

14   See Chapter 13, "Language Development in the Child," in J. Eisenson, I. Ayer, J. Irwin. The Psychology of Communication (New York: Appleton-Century-Crofts, Inc., 1963), for normative data. What expectations should we have of vocabulary acquisition for our two-, three-, and four-year-olds?

more upon words to express his thoughts, ideas, opinions, and wishes. With this dependency on a new skill, the need to be understood becomes an extremely vital part of a child's adjustment and growth. There is no way to estimate the degree of frustration, anxiety, or fear which may be the constant companion of a child whose speech cannot be understood by his playmates, peers, neighbors, or siblings. Fortunately, most mothers can understand the speech of their own children although the child's efforts to communicate may be totally unintelligible to others. Unfortunately, this is not enough.

Although unintelligible speech obviously is ineffective as a communication tool, it is important also to stress that even mildly defective speech can impede communication. For this reason, parents who are anxious about their child's defective speech, often ask: "When should we become concerned about the inaccurate use of speech sounds?" or "What is the expected pattern of speech sound development?"

When parents ask about the development of speech sounds, they usually refer to the development of consonants or what they frequently call "hard sounds." During the process of speech development, a child usually masters consonant sounds in a generally predictive order. By the time an English-speaking child is three

years old, he has acquired the labials or lip sounds (*p, b,* and *m*),
and from three and one-half to four years, the dentals and gutturals
(*t, d, n, k, g,* and *ng*). The labiodentals (*f* and *v*) develop at
about five years of age, and sounds made by complicated tongue
and lip movements (*l, r, zh,* and *ch*) by the sixth year. Other
complicated lip and tongue sounds (*s, z, sh,* and blends such as
st, sl, and *pl*) are usually mastered at the beginning of the seventh
year.

> 15   For a thorough discussion of the development of expressive language
> (speech), see Dorothea McCarthy's chapter, "Language Development in
> Children," in L. Carmichael, ed., *Manual of Child Psychology* (New
> York: John Wiley & Sons, Inc., 1954), pp. 476-581.

From this developmental schedule, it is apparent that a child
of three can be expected to have difficulty with certain sounds
(for example, *l, r,* and *s*), but this speech cannot be considered
defective. If, however, at the age of eight years he still has difficulty
with these same sounds, his speech is defective and should be
evaluated by a speech and hearing specialist. In other words, the
development of a child is considered normal or abnormal depending upon his chronological age and the maturational level of the
particular function being evaluated. The significance of delayed
speech and language development, therefore, changes with time.

USE OF DEVELOPMENTAL SCALES

In recent years, parents have shown an increasingly astute awareness of the various stages of speech and language development.
Mothers in particular frequently spend a significant amount of
time poring over developmental schedules to determine when they
can expect their child's first words. Even after a child begins to
talk, his parents frequently continue to compare his progress with
that of other children his age or with his siblings or with the
averages of the developmental schedules which have become so
popular during the last decade. This interest in developmental

> 16   The popularization of these developmental schedules has been height-
> ened by the magazine and newspaper writings of such well-known
> authorities on child development as Benjamin Spock, Frances Ilg, and
> Louise Ames. A. Gesell, and C. Amatruda, *Developmental Diagnosis*
> (New York: Paul B. Hoeber, Inc., 1947), p. 406; Psyche Cattell, *The
> Measurement of Intelligence of Infants and Young Children* (New York:

The Psychological Corporation, 1947), p. 274, are considered classics by some specialists in child development. Have the norms changed much since these books were written? If so, which items need to be brought up to date?

expectations is necessary for early detection of problems, of course, but certain dangers often accompany this type of awareness and certain warnings seem appropriate.

First, speech does not develop as an isolated skill. No child develops speech without first going through a period of time during which he accumulates knowledge from and about his environment. In essence, a child must *learn* to see, *learn* to hear, *learn* to use his sensory abilities effectively. He must also *learn* pertinent motor patterns—both fine and gross motor skills. The development of mental abilities is also necessary for the development of speech. Hence, not only is speech a learned process, but most of the behavior that forms a basis for speech is also learned. Just as an infant learns first to hold his head erect, to sit alone, and to creep and stand alone, before he is able to take those first wobbly steps prior to walking, speech develops as the result of learned experiences through vision, audition, intelligence, social competence, and nonverbal, as well as verbal, language. Because of this complex interaction of the learning process, parents must be aware of the many factors that form a basis for speech development, and speech must not be considered a skill which develops in isolation or in and of itself.

17 For a challenging discussion of factors involved in the development of speech and language, read Mildred Templin, *Certain Language Skills in Children* (Minneapolis: University of Minnesota Press, 1957).

Second, developmental scales consist of mean scores derived from large samples of behavior, and no single score should be interpreted literally. For example, some children may develop speech much earlier than others. At the same time, these early talkers may not develop as rapidly in other abilities or skills. Conversely, some children may develop speech at a much later date than the mean age which the developmental scale indicates—but they may have developed rather advanced skills in other important behavioral activities, such as walking. It is probably safe to say that no child will develop motor skills, mental abilities, emotional stability, social competence, or speech and language at times suggested as "average" in all of these areas of performance.

Third, because speech does not develop in a vacuum, verbal stimulation is crucial to the development of speech. In fact, speech and language may develop in direct proportion to the kind and amount of verbal stimulation found in the child's environment.

18   An interesting Russian account of differential speech development due to intensive language stimulation of one of two twins is given by A. R. Luria in *Speech and the Development of Mental Processes* (London: Staples Press, 1959). An article by R. W. Howard, "The Language Development of a Group of Triplets," *Journal of Genetic Psychology*, LXIX (1946), pp. 181-88, emphasizes the need for a stimulating verbal environment for language development.

This does not mean that young children should be in a constant whirl of questions, answers, statements, or descriptions, but certainly a child who lives in a world of highly charged meaningful verbal exchanges will have more reason to communicate through speech. Encouraging a child to look at objects and things in his environment, explaining to him the meanings of sounds and noises, helping him to become more sensitive to differences in the way various objects feel, smell, and taste will increase his interest in the world about him and should reinforce his desire to communicate with other people.

Even a normal child will not develop equally in all areas at the same time—some skills will be mastered in advance of the average; others will lag behind. For this reason, one of the most important points to remember in the evaluation of speech and language of young children is the need to consider their speech development against the backdrop of their total development. Only in this way is it possible to differentiate between a problem needing professional attention and one needing additional time for normal maturation. Our task is, of course, to increase our accuracy in detecting problems in young children at the earliest possible time without running the risk of labeling a child as having a problem when actually a problem does not exist.

In order to accomplish this, we must know something about child development, particularly during that period of time from birth to four years. During the first four years, constant change and continuous growth occur in all aspects of development. In fact, never again in life does so much change or so many accomplishments occur in so short a period of time.

THE INFANT (0-1 YEAR)

As early as at one month, an infant gives certain clues as to the social, communicating human being he will eventually become. He has begun, at this early age, to tighten his muscles when he is picked up, and, even though it is only a momentary glance, he will look fleetingly at the person who holds him. He has begun to sort out those things which are pleasant to him and those which are painful or unpleasant. His major mode of communication is crying, and he has just begun to vary his crying as a control of his environment.

He is not, at this stage, a social being, but he makes some random vocal noises which are forerunners of speech and verbal communication. Developmental changes and specific accomplishments during the first three months are remarkable. To the daily observer, each day seems to bring with it a major change, and observing an infant during this period of life is not unlike watching speeded motion pictures of flowers unfolding.

19   The English author, Margaret C. Greene, has written a very pleasant book on speech development in the child as an unfolding process: *Learning to Talk* (New York: Harper & Row, Publishers, 1961).

Thus, at four months the child is well on his way to becoming a social being. He likes to be held, and he delights in being propped up in a sitting position. His motor skills are considerably better at four months than at three. He can follow an object with his eyes and he attempts to reach for objects. When he succeeds in grasping an object, which at this time is very difficult for him, he responds with gurgling and cooing and the unmistakable human response of laughing aloud. When you smile at him, he can smile back at you, and he is fascinated by small pieces of wearing apparel or objects such as pins, buttons, earrings, or glasses—all of which he attempts to grasp, without much success.

His motor development during the next two months is remarkable. At six months he can sit alone with a fair degree of confidence. By seven months, he prefers a sitting position to all others. Regardless of the position he is in, he is content only if he has something in his hand. He explores through the sense of touch. He can sit for unbelievable amounts of time transferring an object from one hand to the other, with, of course, short detours to his mouth. He is friendly and outgoing and smiles at anyone who smiles at him.

Then some rapid changes occur in this friendly, placid, contented human infant. It is during this period from seven to ten

20   For a careful play-by-play account of speech development in the individual child, read *Infant Speech*, by M. M. Lewis (New York: Humanities Press, 1951).

months that the beginnings of the thinking process and language development can be critically observed.

At seven months, for example, a child's awareness and sensitivity have increased to such a degree that he becomes less outgoing and usually shows displeasure with or withdrawal from strangers and strange situations. This beginning of selectiveness emphasizes the fact that he is beginning to express his individuality and is beginning to identify what belongs to his environment and what does not. A child at eight months appears to be less coordinated than previously, but this is because he has so many motor functions partially developed, and both confusion and frustration mark his motor performances.

Then, from nine to ten months comes a brief but welcomed period of organization; he becomes friendly again to his environment, and his sphere of friends appears larger and he usually is socially responsive. One developmental aspect which helps him become a more social being is the fact that he is able to maintain his balance in a sitting position for an indefinite period of time. While doing this, he can amuse himself by manipulating objects. He can also get on his hands and knees in a creeping position. It is during this period of time, therefore, that he begins to learn about space; he learns to creep and move about in his environment.

ONE TO TWO YEARS

At about one year, a child changes from a creeping to a walking animal, and the metamorphosis is more remarkable than just a change in locomotor activity. In the first place, he is no longer restricted to a small amount of space—he has become his "own man," so to speak. The world begins to look different to him. He no longer sees only the bottoms of tables, or the legs of chairs. The floor is no longer his physical focal point. With this new and constantly changing view of the world, language development receives a real boost.

The parents begin to see additional indications of understanding in the child at 15 months. For example, at 15 months a child often uses vocalizations to make known his wants and needs, and he usually reinforces these vocalizations by pointing to the object or thing he desires. He can respond accurately to a few words and phrases, and his protests are made known through body resistance as well as crying, with or without tears.

A child of 18 months can usually be counted upon to do just the opposite of what you ask him to do. If you ask him to "come here," he may stand and look at you, or he may toddle as fast as he can in the opposite direction. If he is holding an object, and you reach your hand out and ask him for it, he usually will throw the object aside or drop it on the floor. He responds to most requests in some way opposite to expectations. Yet, this behavior is not defiance in a child of this age, but rather it may indicate his confusion with *yes* and *no; come* and *go; give* and *take.*

Two to three years

At two years of age, a child is much better organized in every way, and he understands a great amount of what is said to him. He also is able to use words meaningfully, and he no longer depends upon vocalizations and pointing to make his wants known. As he proceeds from two years to three years, he becomes more demanding and more rigid. He is also perseverative—he may continue to perform the same activities over and over again, especially if he can perform these tasks successfully. These are natural developments for a child of this age. If allowed to make a choice, he will usually make it quickly and stick with that decision regardless of what occurs. His decision frequently extends over a long period of time. For example, if allowed to play out of doors on a sunny day, he probably will demand to play outside on a rainy day, refusing or failing to understand the difference. He frequently reacts violently if his plans are interrupted. He demands routine, and it is difficult to introduce new clothes, new toys, or new activities into his everyday living. In terms of language, he has a few pet phrases which he uses constantly. Yet, he is beginning to learn differences in inflection patterns, and he uses these phrases in different ways with different meanings. He knows, for example, the difference between *"mummy* go," indicating that mummy and *only* mummy is to go; "mummy *go,"* stressing that mummy cannot stay; and "mummy go?", which may be one of a long series of questions.

Most parents learn instinctively that the best way to manage a two-and-one-half to three-year-old child is to reduce the number of questions asked him and to make decisions in advance so that he cannot disrupt household routine. It is difficult, under these conditions, to provide the necessary verbal stimulation needed for good language development.

One way to provide speech and language stimulation for a child of this age is by telling him stories at bedtime, a practice which he usually enjoys thoroughly. He may, however, insist that the same stories be told night after night, and if this routine is varied, he may become very unhappy. To some extent, the storyteller might vary the routine by asking questions about story content. This procedure provides an opportunity for introducing new words or new concepts. In this way the child's vocabulary may be extended and enlarged, and other important aspects of learning, such as retention of sequence information, increased memory span, and the development of percepts and concepts can be reinforced.

THREE TO FOUR YEARS

At three years of age the child has temporarily mastered most of the gross motor functions necessary to move around in his environment and some of the fine motor skills needed to manipulate objects. During this period of time, he shows an increased ability with and considerable interest in speech and language. His vocabulary has increased measurably. His ability to understand what is said to him is amazing. Generally speaking, he is an interesting companion and usually a provocative conversationalist. His actions can be controlled by words, to some extent; he usually will stop what he is doing if he hears "No, don't do that." He responds as much to verbal praise as to material reward. He loves new words and may imitate parts of adults' conversation without actually understanding the meaning of the words or phrases. Probably the child who asked, "Where does Gladly, the cross-eyed bear, live?", after hearing the hymn "Gladly the Cross I'd Bear," was in this general age group. The three-year-old also enjoys special words with mysterious or different meanings. Complete cooperation is almost assured through sincere promises of "I'm going to tell you a secret," or "We are going to play a game of magic," or "Tomorrow we are going to have a surprise."

As a child approaches four years of age, much of the coordination he has maintained in the past becomes disrupted, and he may become awkward or generally poorly coordinated. Hesitations in speech patterns may also be heard at this time, and the child may be uncertain in the same speech situations that he appeared to have mastered just previously. For this reason, many parents become alarmed about their child's speech and language during this developmental period.

At times, a child may show some regression in communication; he may seem confused, anxious, and even less alert than he appeared previously. This can be the result of parental demands that he perform consistently and accurately on all tasks, some of which may be above his maturation level. Again, this is a reminder that a child does not develop constantly or consistently in all areas of performance simultaneously, and the straight-line graphs of developmental charts which have been based on general averages may be deceiving in this respect. Actually, periods of plateau in development are to be expected, because a child, like everyone else, must absorb what he has learned before the task is actually mastered.

This brief, cursory discussion of some of the developmental highlights during the first four years of life is intended to serve at least one major purpose: to emphasize that speech and language acquisition, although vital to this period of growth, is just one phase of a child's total development, and that the evaluation of speech and language, if it is to be meaningful, must be viewed against a backdrop of all other spheres of development, including the motor, sensory, intellectual, social, and emotional modalities. This point, although recognized academically by those professionally concerned with speech and language disorders, frequently becomes obscured during the evaluation of a child who is delayed in speech development, particularly when speech is viewed as an isolated process rather than as part of the total developmental sequence.

Because of the many skills which must be mastered and the many kinds of information which must be absorbed and learned during early childhood, professional observers of speech and language development usually are not amazed at the frequency with which delayed speech and language occurs in childhood. To the contrary, after considering the many facets of the child which must develop simultaneously, and being aware of the complexity of the communication process, it seems to them more astonishing that so many children develop speech without complication. This point becomes even more cogent as we consider the numerous factors which can impede and delay the development of speech and language.

AT THE OUTSET OF ANY DISCUSSION OF CAUSAL FACTORS ASSOCIATED with delayed speech and language development, certain points concerning the detection of causes should be considered.

First, some causes of delayed speech and language are not known, and others are not understood completely. Therefore, in some cases, the cause cannot be determined even when the most valid and reliable diagnostic procedures are used, and even when the examiners are known to be well skilled in administering these tests. But these cases are in the minority, and the fact that they exist should not serve to relax our efforts in the detection of cause nor should they be considered an excuse to accept a less-than-satisfactory exploration of the problem.

Second, at times more than one factor is reported as the cause for

2 causal factors of delayed speech and language development

a child's delayed speech and language development. Like the blind men who attempted to describe an elephant each by taking hold of a different part of the animal, specialists from different disciplines may have different opinions as to the cause or causes of a child's delayed speech. However, each of these specialists may be correct in his statement of cause, for multiple problems may be present, each acting as an impeding factor in speech and language development.

Third, available methods for measuring the degree of speech and language delay frequently are not inclusive enough or incisive enough to incorporate all of the many dimensions which should be considered in determining the degree of delay. In some cases, therefore, we are limited to giving subjective opinions or judgments as to the degree of delayed speech, using nonspecific terms such as: *mild, moderate,* or *severe* to describe how much delay is present. Nevertheless, every effort should be made to devise objective measurements to evaluate objectively those dimensions of speech and language which currently must be evaluated subjectively.

These points emphasize the importance of tracing the cause or causes of delayed speech and language and the need for estimating, as objectively as possible, the degree to which the delay exists. Even more critically, they emphasize our need to have a clear conception of what we mean by the term *delayed speech.*

What *do* we mean when we say that a child has delayed speech? Do we mean that his speech is delayed permanently and that he may never be able to use speech effectively? Or do we mean that his speech delay is temporary and that, with help, he may be able to develop normal speech? Do we mean that his speech development is delayed only to a minor degree, and that he will need only minimum help with his problem? Or do we mean that he has a moderate to severe disorder, which may not be remedial but which will require concentrated help over a relatively long period of time? Do we mean that a speech and hearing specialist is the best source of help for his problem? Or does our use of the term imply that he will need help from various disciplines, in both the evaluation and the treatment of his problem? These are just a few of the possible implications of the term *delayed speech,* and it is understandable, therefore, why confusion surrounds the use of it.

21   For a discussion of this term and some of its implications, read Chapter 6, "Delayed Speech," in C. Van Riper, *Speech Correction: Principles and Methods* (Englewood Cliffs, N.J.: Prentice-Hall, Inc., 1963), pp. 102-31.

At best, the term *delayed speech* is a broad classification which refers only to the fact that a child has not acquired speech at the expected time nor with the expected accuracy. It is not, and should not be considered, a diagnostic term, for it indicates nothing about the cause of speech delay, the degree to which the problem exists, or the extent to which the problem might be alleviated or measurably reduced.

Perhaps one way to strengthen the significance and the clinical use of the term *delayed speech* is to link the intended meaning of the term, as closely as possible, with the cause or causes of the speech and language delay. In this way, the diagnostic sequence, of which the detection of cause is one part, would have at least two major purposes: to ascertain, if possible, what has caused the speech and language delay, and to determine, in general, to what degree the delay exists. This, of course, is not a simple procedure.

The causes of delayed speech and language development are viewed most frequently from two standpoints: as those problems stemming from *organic* involvement, and as those nonorganic factors which, perhaps for lack of a more precise term, are called *functional* problems. Still another way of viewing causes of delayed

22   Margaret H. Powers speaks of the inadequacy of this term in her two
chapters concerning articulation disorders in *The Handbook of Speech
Pathology*, L. E. Travis, ed. (New York: Appleton-Century-Crofts, Inc.,
1957), pp. 707-804.

speech and language development, and the way in which causes will be discussed here, is to consider what is needed for adequate speech and language development and then to consider what problems can interrupt or impede this process.

Adequate speech and language develops as a result of a fortunate combination of factors. Integrity of the central nervous system, adequate mental abilities, well-functioning sensory pathways, emotional stability, a stimulating speech environment, and adequate maturation are all needed for normal speech and language development. Hence, speech and language development can be delayed permanently, or impeded temporarily, by problems associated with central nervous system impairment, mental retardation, hearing loss, emotional disturbance, environmental deprivation, or immaturity. These various disorders may occur either separately or in combination.

CENTRAL NERVOUS SYSTEM IMPAIRMENT

The central nervous system is more complex and more mysterious in the way it works than all the man-developed computers and other man-made informational systems put together. Our attempts to understand more about the central nervous system and the way in which the brain works have been advanced measurably during the last decade, but our knowledge is still very primitive.

All of the higher brain functions of man, such as symbol organization, judgment of relationships, attention and concentration, percept and concept formation, cognition, inductive and deductive reasoning, control of impulse, visual and auditory memory, recall and recognition, and the perceptual motor processes are dependent upon the integrity of the central nervous system. Therefore, certain behavioral deviations, as well as language disorders and learning disabilities, can result from central nervous system impairment. Frequently these deviations, disorders, and disabilities occur in the absence of specific signs of neurologic impairment or mental retardation. Neurologists are faced with a formidable task when they undertake the formal neurologic examination of young children. The procedures are complicated to an even greater degree if the child cannot talk and if no apparent neurologic signs of a central nervous system disorder are present. Yet, even in the absence of obvious neurologic signs, a neurologist may observe clinical clues which support his diagnosis of cerebral dysfunction. To express this clinical opinion, the term *minimal brain damage* has been used to indicate that a central nervous system disorder is present.

> 23   Unfortunately, this term has been used indiscriminately to describe children with certain types of deviant behavior, sometimes without benefit of neurologic examination or medical evidence. For an excellent discussion of "minimal brain damage," see the article by Raymond L. Clemmens, M.D., "Minimal Brain Damage in Children," in *Children*, VIII, No. 5, 179-83. Another discussion along this dimension can be found in Knobloch and Pasamanick's article, "Syndrome of Minimal Cerebral Damage in Infancy," in the *Journal of the American Medical Association*, CLXX (1959), 384.

The recently popular emphasis on organic disorders has created some problems in the interpretation of information to parents. One of the areas of danger lies in the use of medical terminology by nonmedical specialists. Frequently the interpretation to parents of the results of the total examination becomes the responsibility of the psychologist, speech pathologist, or teacher. With this responsibility, it is important to see that considerable care is taken in the interpretation of clinical findings, to require that findings be substantiated clearly by the fact, and to avoid contributing to parental anxiety, which sometimes is thus created needlessly.

Some of the dangers involved in the indiscriminate use of terminology can be seen in the following clinical example. Mark, a three-year-old boy, was referred to a clinic for examination because he had not developed speech and was unable to communicate his wants and needs to others. His parents reported that he had severe temper tantrums at home and that frequently this behavior did not appear to be related to circumstances in the environment nor were they predictable. They reported also that he was hyperactive and extremely difficult to manage. Psychologic examinations indicated that he was not mentally retarded or emotionally disturbed. The referral report from the pediatrician indicated that Mark was physically normal and that he gave evidence of being able to hear.

Further audiologic examinations supported the fact that Mark could hear, but the report indicated that he was unable to or refused to make practical or social use of his hearing. However, on the isolated basis of Mark's hyperactivity and the difficulties involved in managing him, both at home and in a clinical setting, the therapist assigned to work with him inserted in his case history report that he was "apparently" *minimally brain damaged.* Fortunately in this case, the report of minimal brain damage was not interpreted to the child's parents, for subsequent testing revealed that there was no neurologic evidence to support such a statement, and formal neurologic tests negated the possibility that such a problem existed.

The lesson to be learned from the foregoing example is a crucial one: each specialist must stick to his specialty. Although the search for the cause of the problem is always an important and continuing investigation, a clinical classification which is not supported by facts, or terminology which has been lifted from another profession and used with little or no professional competence, can be both dangerous and impeding to the effective handling of the problem. It is one thing for specialists to understand the terminology used by other professional disciplines; it is another for them to adopt this terminology, using it out of context and with little knowledge of the implications of the terms. This is an extremely important point to remember throughout the following discussion.

BEHAVIORAL CLUES ASSOCIATED WITH
CENTRAL NERVOUS SYSTEM IMPAIRMENT

Disturbances in behavior associated with brain damage provide vital diagnostic clues even in the absence of notable neurologic signs. Behavioral clues, such as hyperactivity, perseveration, distractibility, catastrophic behavior, visual-motor disturbance, and figure-ground disorders usually are called organic behavior disorders.

24 Behavioral manifestations associated with central nervous system impairment are discussed in articles which have been noted in Search Item 23. In addition to these references, also read C. Bradley's discussion, "Characteristics and Management of Children with Behavior Problems Associated with Organic Brain Damage," in *The Pediatric Clinics of North America,* I (November 1957), 1949-1960, and P. J. Doyle's "The Organic Hyperkinetic Syndrome," *The Journal of School Health,* XXXII (October 1962), No. 8.

These organic behavior disorders are accompanied often by other problems; language disorders and learning disabilities are two types of problems which occur frequently. When language disorders and learning disabilities are associated with brain damage, they are referred to frequently as *psychoneurological learning disorders*. The term *neuropsychiatric learning disorders* may be used also, depending, apparently, on the area of specialty (psychology or neurology) represented by the person responsible for using the term.

25 See "Psychoneurological Learning Disorders in Children," by H. R. Myklebust and B. Boshes, published in *Archives of Pediatrics* (June 1960), 247-56. Neuropsychiatric learning disorders are discussed in an article by R. L. Clemmens, "Minimal Brain Damage in Children," *Children*, VIII No. 5, 179-83. For additional information, the interested student may wish to refer to H. F. Burks' discussion, "The Effect of Brain Pathology on Learning," in *Exceptional Children*, XXIV (1957) 169-72, and to A. J. Yates' article, "Disorders of Speech, Brain Damage and Learning Theory," *Education*, LXXIX (1959), No. 7, 444-47.

Hyperactivity and distractibility are noted frequently in children with central nervous system impairment; random wanderings and short attention span are major components of the behavior of these children. As a consequence of his hyperactivity and his constant distraction, the quality of such a child's performance on tasks requiring motor skills or mental abilities is usually poor. This is due to the fact that these children are unable consistently to ignore the numerous irrelevant stimuli within their environment. Much of what is distracting to these children is screened out early and selectively by normal children. This "forced responsiveness" suggests strongly that these children need to attend to all stimuli with equal attention, and that they are forced to attend without control and without any real intention to their response.

In keeping with this absence of control or intention, a brain-damaged child's behavior may take on a general bizarre character, the nature of which clearly indicates that he has reason for his unpredictable, disorganized, and disrupted behavior. This inability to control responses has been described as "organic driven-ness," a term which indicates that energies are driven from within, without the normal controls that are usually superimposed on such responses.

26 More information about the effects of hyperkinetic behavior and distractibility can be found in "Hyperkinetic Behavior Syndrome in Children," *The Journal of Pediatrics*, L (April 1957), 463-74, by M. W.

Laufer, and in "The Hyperkinetic Impulse Disorder in Children's Behavior Problems," *Psychosomatic Medicine,* XIX (1957), 463-74, by
Laufer, Denhoff, and Solomons. It is important to consider what effects
hyperkinetic behavior may have on learning. For some idea about this,
read Burks' "The Hyperkinetic Child," in *Exceptional Children,* XXVII
(September 1960), 18-26.

Although central nervous system impairment is known to be one
of the causes of delayed speech and language development, current
detection methods used to diagnose central nervous system impairment in young children are not refined enough to state with absolute certainty that damage to the central nervous system does or
does not exist. This is true particularly when behavioral clues,
some of which have been discussed previously, cannot be identified
clearly or when it is questionable whether such responses are indicative of deviant behavior. The point is: hyperactivity and perseverative behavior are seen frequently in normal children. For example,
at two and three years of age, a child might spend much of
his time exploring his new world and testing his environment in a
rather random manner. Yet, with all of his random exploration, his
flitting about the room, his short attention span, and the difficulty
his parents may experience in controlling him, his behavior is not
considered deviant. And when he finds something which intrigues
him, a young child may continue to explore a particular object or
thing for a long, seemingly endless period of time. In fact, much of
the exploration which is carried out at this age is continued well
past the time which might seem appropriate. However, when he
becomes unduly concerned with one activity, his behavior is not
considered perseverative. In a young child of two or three years,
both hyperactivity and perseveration are considered acceptable behavior. Conversely, this very same behavior in an older child of
six or seven, in the same settings, may be classified as hyperactivity
or perseveration. Thus, one dimension along which behavior can
be considered deviant or not is the appropriateness of the behavior
to the age of the child.

Some clues to the diagnosis of central nervous systems impairment are overt entirely and not difficult to link with specific etiologies. When motor incapacity or severe incoordination is present,
as seen, for example, in children with cerebral palsy, the cause is
not difficult to detect, because the physical characteristics are linked
conclusively with brain damage. However, in a child where the

electroencephalogram is not positive, or where other physical characteristics which can be causally linked with impairment of the central nervous system are not present, the behavior of the child may be the only way to identify and isolate causal factors. It is for this reason that the observation of behavior, by specialists trained to recognize subtle clues and with experience enough to associate these clues accurately with causal factors, is a major source of information in the differential diagnosis of organic disorders in young children.

27   For a case study of a "brain-injured child," see pages 107-9 of this text, and for an interesting account of behavioral clues associated with brain damage, see Milman's "Organic Brain Disorder: Behavior Characteristics of Brain Damaged Children," AMA American Journal of Diseases of Children, XCI (1956), 521-28. Compare these characteristics with those found in Bradley's "Organic Factors in the Psychopathology of Childhood," in H. P. Hoch, ed., Psychopathology of Childhood (New York: Grune & Stratton, Inc., 1955), pp. 82-103.

LANGUAGE DISORDERS ASSOCIATED WITH CENTRAL NERVOUS SYSTEM IMPAIRMENT

There are few, if any, speech and hearing specialists who have not been faced with the problem of providing adequate service for children with language disorders. State directors of special education and supervisors of speech and hearing services have reported increasing numbers of requests for help for these children in recent years. University clinics and community centers designed to offer diagnostic services for children and adults with language disabilities find that measurably larger numbers of children are being referred for evaluation than in the past. While educators throughout the nation are seeking effective methods for teaching these children, the parents seem almost frantic in their attempts to locate programs which will accept their child and understand his problem.

Language disorders is a broad term which refers to the inability or limited ability of an individual to use linguistic symbols for communication. The term, therefore, includes disorders of reading and writing, as well as speaking. *Aphasia* refers to difficulty in the comprehension and use of linguistic symbols for *oral* communication, whereas the term *alexia* is used to describe disorders of *reading*,

ρ dysgraphia

and *agraphia* is used to describe disorders of *writing*. Some specialists prefer the terms *dysphasia, dyslexia,* and *dysgraphia* to indicate central problems in speech, reading, and writing, respectively. The change in prefix is used to designate a partial, rather than total, problem.

> 28   These terms are described and defined in numerous writings, including H. Myklebust's "Language Disorders in Children," *Exceptional Children,* XXII (January 1956), No. 4, 163-66. For further discussion of these terms, two monographs on the subject by N. Wood may be of some help: *Language Development and Language Disorders: A Compendium of Lectures* (Child Development Publications of the Society for Research in Child Development, Inc., April 1960), and *Language Disorders in Children* (Chicago: National Society for Crippled Children and Adults, 1959).

In the past, arguments have been presented against the use of the term *congenital* as an adjective to describe language disorders in young children, on the basis that language disorders cannot be present at birth. The argument is that, because speaking, reading, and writing are not possible at birth, and because instead of losing these abilities the child has never acquired them, they cannot be considered *congenital* problems. On the other side of the coin, those who believe that aphasia *can* be a congenital problem argue that, when central nervous system impairment occurs during or immediately following birth, a predisposition or predilection toward a language disorder or a learning disability is present at birth, and, therefore, the resulting problem can be classified as congenital.

> 29   The essence of both sides of this argument can be reviewed by reading two monographs: *The Concept of Congenital Aphasia from the Standpoint of Dynamic Differential Diagnosis* (Washington, D. C.: American Speech and Hearing Association, 1959); and *Childhood Aphasia: Proceedings of the Institute of Childhood Aphasia* (San Francisco, Calif.: Gillick Printing, Inc., 1952).

Some specialists consider language disorders in children to be developmental problems, some of which are thought to be transitory. In addition, there are *acquired* cases of language disorders, which occur when the child has been able to speak, read, and write but has lost one or all of these abilities when injury to the central nervous system has occurred through accident or some other kind of trauma.

30   For a discussion of developmental aphasia, see M. E. Morley's discus-
      sion, "Delayed Speech and Developmental Aphasia," in the *British
      Medical Journal,* II (1955), 463-67. Information concerning acquired
      aphasia can be found in M. E. Manteno's and J. Hazon's article,
      "Acquired Aphasia in Children," found in *Pediatric Americana,* III
      (1945), 188-92.

APHASIA

The term *aphasia* is often defined as a lack or partial lack of
speech resulting from injury to the brain. Realistically, the problem
is much more complex. More accurately, aphasia in children refers

31   This complexity is discussed from various viewpoints in the March 1959
      edition of *Education,* which is devoted entirely to a discussion of lan-
      guage disorders in children. Read A. L. Benton's article in that issue,
      "Aphasia in Children," pp. 408-12.

to the child's inability to use symbols for communication. Therefore, a child with aphasia is unable to comprehend or use speech
for communication because he is unable to understand the meaning
of *verbal symbols* (that is, words). It has been said that a child with
aphasia responds in much the same way that a normal-speaking
person might in a country where the natives speak a language entirely foreign to the visitor. This analogy, however, falls far short
of describing the problem of aphasia. Not only is the aphasic child
surrounded by a language which he cannot understand but, equally
important, few people recognize that he does not understand speech
and cannot comprehend words. He has no interpreters, no way to
make his wants known. And, because he has a learning problem,
he cannot learn to speak by listening to others talk. Unlike the
normal-speaking person traveling in a foreign country, the child
with aphasia has no country he calls his own — at least, from a language standpoint. Because of his communication barrier, observers
may think that he is mentally retarded, or deaf, or emotionally disturbed, and they respond to him in terms of whichever problem
they think they have identified. Yet, the child with aphasia differs
markedly from children with delayed speech and language development resulting from other disorders. As we will discuss in more
detail later, a deaf child does not develop speech normally, but his
lack of speech development is related directly to his inability to
hear sound. A mentally retarded child does not develop speech

normally, but his inability to comprehend or use verbal symbols is not his only area of deficiency. An emotionally disturbed child may not develop any speech, owing possibly to his rejection of words, but his problem is not considered a disturbance in symbolic formulation. Diagnostically, these differentiations are of extreme importance, and numerous specialists have devoted considerable effort toward the differential diagnosis of aphasia in children.

32 For a discussion of various points of view, read *Childhood Aphasia Proceedings*, R. West, ed. (San Francisco, Calif.: Gillick Printing, Inc., 1962).

The development of normal language depends upon the reception and integration of incoming stimuli before the expression of language can logically follow. Functionally, language can be divided into three types: *expressive language*, or the language used to communicate with others (speaking and writing); *receptive language*, or the language used to understand what others say (reading and listening); *integrative language*, or the language used internally for thinking or reflection. Children with aphasia are usually classified as having a primary problem at one of these three levels of communication. It is, however, unusual for a child to have a problem that is entirely expressive, unless some *dyspraxia* is present. Usually, a child with aphasia has a *mixed* problem and shows evidence of limited expressive language and a reduced ability to understand or comprehend language symbols. If a severe problem exists, such as a gross lack of language development or a severe inner language involvement, the problem may be classified as *central aphasia*. The distinguishing difference between central aphasia and mental deficiency is the indication by psychologic tests that the intellectual potential of the child with aphasia is considerably higher than his actual performance level. This higher potential is not present in the mentally deficient child.

33 For an interdisciplinary approach to the study of aphasia read C. E. Osgood and M. S. Miron, *Approaches to the Study of Aphasia* (Urbana, Illinois: University of Illinois Press, 1963), p. 210. This book is the result of a research seminar concerned with aphasia where specialists and authorities on the subject discussed normal language production, the definition of aphasia, components of the disorder, concomitant behavior, lesions producing disabilities, and recovery from aphasia.

Unquestionably, the diagnostic aspects of aphasia in children are complex, requiring the combined attention of specialists from various disciplines. For example, because of the complexity of evaluation, neurologists, pediatricians, otologists, psychologists, audiologists, and speech and language pathologists are only a few of the specialists who may be concerned with the differential diagnosis of aphasia in children. In general, at least four major points in the basic differentiation of aphasia from other problems should be noted:

First, the classification of aphasia in children assumes that the major factor separating this disorder from all other speech and language problems is the disturbance in symbolic language formulation. As we mentioned previously, the deaf child does not develop speech normally, but his lack of speech production is related directly to his inability to hear sound. Yet deaf children may have integrated symbolic language in all language functions that do not require sound. The mentally retarded child functions at a retarded symbolic level, but symbolic formulation is not the only area of his deficiency. Thus, the mentally retarded child is expected to develop symbolic language in proportion to his mental age. The emotionally disturbed child may reject sound and may not talk, but his problem, again, is not relegated to a primary disturbance in symbolic formulation. Diagnostically, these differentiations are of extreme importance.

Second, some of the more overt symptoms of aphasia may resemble the symptoms of other childhood problems, but the total problem constellations are distinctly different. The mentally deficient child may have some abilities in which he is more proficient than others, but the general index of his performance indicates permanent retardation in all areas. Although the aphasic child may resemble the mentally retarded child because of an inability to perform adequately on standardized intelligence tests, the abilities

34   This contrast is discussed in more detail by M. J. Berko in "Mental
      Evaluation of the Aphasic Child," *American Journal of Occupational
      Therapy*, V (1951), No. 6, and by I. W. Karlin in "Aphasias in Chil-
      dren," *American Journal of Disabled Children*, LXXXVII (1954), 752.

involved — not the degree of retardation — is the important differentiating factor. The deaf child, because of his inability to hear sound, is unable to perform tests which require hearing for adequate performance. The aphasic child may resemble the deaf child because of fluctuating responses to sound, but the differentiating factor is that the aphasic child has a normal hearing mechanism. The emotionally disturbed child has specific types of bizarre behavior which often render him socially inadequate. Although the aphasic child and the emotionally disturbed child may be confused diagnostically because both may have behavior problems, the behavior patterns of the child with aphasia are related to his communication disorder, caused by cortical damage. Therefore, disturbed behavior must be analyzed with reference to the cause of the disturbance if habilitative planning is to meet the needs of the problem.

Third, the classification of aphasia cannot be used merely because all other possible diagnostic classifications have been excluded. If, in the diagnostic evaluation of a nonverbal child, he is found *not* to be mentally retarded, *not* to be deaf, and *not* to be emotionally disturbed, it is important to emphasize also that he may *not* be aphasic. The diagnosis of the nonverbal child is not advanced enough at the present time, nor, perhaps, will it ever be, to use such a process of elimination with finality. Because there are many reasons for delayed speech of which we are not aware, unless the child has a symbolic formulation disorder, his problem cannot be classified as aphasia.

Fourth, a child with aphasia requires an educational approach that is designed for his particular problem, and educational processes currently used for children with mental retardation, emotional disturbance, or deafness will not produce maximum results. The

35 For more information concerning this point, read W. C. Barger, "Experimental Approach to Aphasic and Nonreading Children," *American Journal of Orthopsychiatry*, XXIII (1953), 158; A. McGinnis, and others, *Teaching Aphasic Children* (Washington, D. C.: The Volta Bureau, Reprint No. 677); H. R. Myklebust, *Training Aphasic Children* (Washington, D. C.: The Volta Bureau, Reprint No. 660); and N. Wood, "Language Disorders: An Educational Problem," *Education*, CCCXCIX (1959), 79.

mentally retarded child, because of the permanent nature of his problem, requires *simplification, drill,* and *repetition* in order to retain basic educational principles. The emotionally disturbed child is usually seen in a *permissive* atmosphere with a psychoanalytic orientation. The deaf child requires auditory training and speech reading, with specific educational procedures that are designed to help him *compensate* for his hearing loss. The aphasic child must be helped to *organize* incoming stimuli so that they can be used more meaningfully for communication purposes.

Therefore, because the aphasic child has specific educational needs, it is considered unwise to place him in educational programs designed for children with other problems. In fact, to do so is detrimental not only to the child with aphasia but also to the other children who are correctly placed in programs designed for their particular problems.

Various programs with different approaches have been designed for the education of the child with aphasia.

36   See A. McGinnis and others, *Teaching Aphasic Children* (Washington, D. C.: The Volta Bureau, Reprint No. 677); H. R. Myklebust, *Training Aphasic Children* (Washington, D. C.: The Volta Bureau, Reprint No. 660); and M. F. Palmer and F. Berko, "Education of the Aphasic Child," *American Journal of Occupational Therapy*, VI (1952), 6.

Regardless of differences in approach or setting, most professional people concerned with the aphasic child agree that he needs a specialized program. In such a program, parent-child relationships are of significant importance. Therefore, it remains the responsi-

37   D. McCarthy discusses these relationships in "Language Disorders and Parent-Child Relationships," *Journal of Speech and Hearing Disorders*, XIX (1954), 514.

bility of the physician, psychologist, speech pathologist, special education teachers, and others to provide the necessary knowledge, facilities, and personnel for the education of the child with aphasia.

Briefly, aphasia in children refers to the child's inability or severely limited ability to use symbols for communication. Differential diagnosis of aphasia is a complex process which requires the services of many different professional disciplines. Although the symptoms of aphasia may resemble those observed in children with mental retardation, an emotional disturbance, or deafness, the causal factors are significantly different. For this reason, aphasic children cannot learn adequately in programs designed for children with other problems. Progress has been made in the classification and identification of aphasia in children, but additional knowledge, facilities, and professional personnel are needed in order to provide for the education of these children.

DYSARTHRIA AND DYSPRAXIA

Dysarthria and dyspraxia can also contribute to delayed speech development and language development. When used to describe a speech disorder, the term *dysarthria* refers to a severe motor problem of the jaw and tongue. Associated with central nervous system impairment, dysarthria is typically observed in children with cerebral palsy. However, dysarthria can occur also in individuals who have no obvious involvement of the arms and legs. It can be present as an isolated problem, and in all degrees of impairment from mild to severe. Children with dysarthria are unable to control the fine jaw or tongue movements necessary for speech, which, when dysarthria is present, is slurred and frequently unintelligible. These children talk as if the entire length of their tongue were rooted to the floor of their mouth. Not only is the child with dysarthria unable to move his lower jaw and tongue independently when he wants to or when requested to do so, but he is unable to use his tongue and jaws adequately for chewing or eating. Swallowing is difficult for him, also.

Dysarthria should not be confused with dyspraxia, although the symptoms are similar in both problems. In dyspraxia, however, the difficulty occurs when the child attempts to perform certain motor functions with his tongue or jaw *voluntarily*. Opening and closing his mouth on command and lifting, protruding or moving his tongue back and forth laterally when requested are difficult, if not impossible, for him. He may, however, be able to perform these motor skills on an *involuntary* basis with ease, particularly when these motor skills are part of other involuntary motor activities, such as eating, licking the lips, or swallowing food or drink.

Dysarthria, then, refers to an inability to perform certain motor functions because of impairment to the motor function itself, as seen in paralysis. Dyspraxia refers to the inability of the individual to associate or recall motor patterns in order to know what must be done to perform a specific motor function. A child with dyspraxia, therefore, has little or no direct control over the organs of speech, although there is nothing organically wrong with them.

38   For additional information about the differentiation between dysarthria
      and dyspraxia, read E. Froeschels, *Dysarthric Speech* (Magnolia, Mass.:
      Expression Company, 1952), and M. E. Morley *et al.*, "Developmental
      dysarthria," *British Medical Journal*, I (1954), 8-10.

MENTAL RETARDATION

One of the most difficult decisions in determining the cause of
delayed speech and language development involves the separation
of other problems from that of mental retardation. Actually, the
term *mental retardation* has become a rather ill-defined, nebulous
designation which gives no indication of the degree of mental subnormality, the causes of the problem, or the prognostic implications. Yet, the term is used by both professional personnel and
laymen.

39   For an exhaustive review of research pertaining to mental subnormality,
      see Richard L. Masland, Seymour B. Sarason, and Thomas Gladwin,
      Mental Subnormality: Biological, Psychological, and Cultural Factors
      (New York: Basic Books, Inc., 1959), pp. 3-439.

If we define *mental retardation* as a reduced mental capacity in
all functions that are basic to learning, a mentally retarded child
would be expected to be delayed in the acquisition of speech and
language as well as in other learned functions. Conversely, if a
child is delayed in the acquisition of speech and language for reasons other than mental retardation, it can be assumed that he
should function at a normal or near-normal level on test items
which do not examine him in his special area of deficiency. Basically, these normal capacities should make it possible for children
who are *not* mentally retarded to compensate, at least partially, for
their communication disorders. For this reason, children with such
problems as aphasia, hearing loss, or emotional disturbance must
be considered different from normal children in *kind* rather than
degree, whereas the mentally retarded child is different in *degree*
rather than *kind*. Stated differently, a mentally retarded child has
a reduced ability to learn adequately from *any* experience within
his environment, whereas children with aphasia, hearing loss, or
emotional disturbance are able to learn from *certain types* of experience, depending upon their individual problems.

When mental retardation is severe, it can be differentiated from
other disorders with a fair degree of certainty. It is difficult, how-

ever, to make this clinical differentiation in children with complex communication disorders. Because tests of mental ability require communication between child and examiner, the communication problem by itself could result in an erroneous diagnosis of mental retardation. Before a child is classified as mentally retarded, considerable supportive evidence must be obtained and every possible avenue of the child's potential must be explored, to be sure that the problem *is* mental retardation and not some other which might be remedied to some extent if accurately diagnosed.

40   This point is stressed further in N. Wood, "Causal Factors of Delayed Speech and Language Development," *American Journal on Mental Deficiency,* LXI (1957), 4. Also see *Proceedings of the 1959 Annual Meeting of the Association for the Aid of Crippled Children: The Child with Brain Damage* (New York: Association for the Aid of Crippled Children, 1961), pp. 4-23, for additional information concerning the need for exhaustive testing procedures when mental retardation is suspected.

Certain behavioral patterns and responses are expected from the mentally retarded child. For example, in addition to being severely delayed in the acquisition of speech and language, he is usually slower in developing motor skills, unable to learn basic subjects in school, and limited in both concrete and abstract thinking. Mental retardation can be caused by a variety of factors: chromosome imbalance (for example, Down's Syndrome or mongolism); damage to the central nervous system (for example, anoxia in premature births), and familial or constitutional problems, among other factors.

Considerable medical advances have been made through studies of genetic disorders and biochemical imbalances. The child who is

41   See the report of the President's Panel on Mental Retardation, *A Proposed Program for National Action to Combat Mental Retardation* (Washington, D. C.: U. S. Government Printing Office, 1963), p. 201.

mentally retarded as the result of cerebral damage, however, presents a complicated picture and requires a complex evaluation. Unlike the child whose mental subnormality stems from genetic, familial, or biochemical causes, the child with central nervous system impairment may not respond at a consistently lowered intellectual level in all areas. In fact, the quintessence of the brain-damaged retardate is "inconsistency," not only in his varying abilities but in his day-to-day performance of activities in which he is known to be competent. For this reason, no single evaluation is able to tap the many facets of the mentally retarded child whose mental subnormality results from cerebral damage.

> 42   The relationship of brain injury to delayed and defective speech is described in detail by Schlanger in Chapter XV of Levin, *Voice and Speech Disorders: Medical Aspects* (Springfield, Ill.: Charles C. Thomas, Publisher, 1962). Also see James J. Gallagher, E. Paul Benoit and Herbert F. Boyd, "Measures of Intelligence in Brain Damaged Children," *Journal of Clinical Psychology,* VII (January 1956), No. 1, 69-72.

As we have said, some children are mentally subnormal as the result of genetic, familial, or biochemical causes. These are considered to be *endogenous* factors, meaning that the problem comes from "within the genes." Others, destined to be normal children, are mentally retarded as the result of injury to the central nervous system, or due to some other trauma, which interrupts normal development. These factors are called *exogenous,* meaning "outside the genes." Regardless of the cause, the problem of mental retardation probably occurs more frequently and creates more parental anxiety than any other childhood disorder.

Although delayed speech and language development might be caused by mental retardation, the cause must be studied in terms of each child's strengths and weaknesses, his abilities and disabilities. First, we must determine how the child *does* communicate. Often we are so busy finding things *wrong* with the communication attempts of a child known to be mentally subnormal, that we fail to consider what is *right* with his communication. Because we are concerned with his inadequacies, we miss what he is telling us when he uses gestures, or points, or expresses himself with body movements or single words.

> 43   For a comprehensive discussion of speech problems of the mentally retarded, see Chapter XVII, written by J. Mathews, in *The Handbook of Speech Pathology,* L. E. Travis, ed. (New York: Appleton-Century-Crofts, Inc., 1957), pp. 531-52.

Second, we must determine at what level a child *is* functioning and what his potential performance level might be for any given task. General assumptions should not be made about children with mental retardation, for each child is a separate entity, with separate problems and varying degrees of retardation.

At times, our educational aspirations for a mentally retarded child may be too high and generally unrealistic. By placing these children in an environment of stress, additional problems may be triggered, resulting in erratic responses, bizarre behavior, social distress, or emotional disturbance. Just as frequently, our expectations may be too low. In these cases, we fail to require enough of the child, so that he continues to function at a level considerably below his potential level.

44 *Educating the Retarded Child* (Boston: Houghton Mifflin Company, 1951), written by S. A. Kirk and G. O. Johnson, is a comprehensive treatment of the education of the retarded child and the many complexities that both teachers and parents face in planning an educational program for these children.

Third, we must attempt to determine what problems other than mental retardation are present. In some ways, mental retardation is like fever — it accompanies, or is accompanied by, a number of problems. Therefore, in addition to mental retardation, a child may have seizures, a hearing loss, an emotional problem, aphasia, environmental deprivation, and so forth. Because all of these factors play a part in the child's inability to function adequately, each aspect must be considered separately in terms of possible cause.

45 See B. Schlanger's discussion of other factors which may cloud the picture of mental retardation in "Mentally Retarded and/or Aphasic," *Training School Bulletin,* LX (February 1958), 62-65.

Mental retardation has many facets which require the attention of various professional and allied professional personnel, all of whom play an important role in determining the causes, treatment needs, educability, and potential level of performance of a mentally retarded child, because one of the major components of mental retardation is delayed speech and language development.

Briefly, the mentally retarded child's communication disability lies basically in his inadequate language development, which, as indicated previously, may be caused by either organic or nonorganic factors. The determination of the cause of the problem is important for therapeutic and educational planning.

46 For a description of a mentally retarded child, see pages 117-18 in this text. Other case studies of mentally retarded children can be found in R. Masland, S. Sarason, and T. Gladwin, *Mental Subnormality* (New York: Basic Books, Inc., 1958), pp. 311-58.

EMOTIONAL DISTURBANCE

Emotional stability is not achieved in isolation. Rather, it develops as an integral part of the child's total physical, intellectual, and social development. Generally speaking, a child who is thought of as normal in terms of emotional development is one who is in harmony with himself and with his environment. In essence, he is a child who conforms to the emotional and social requirements of his culture. Although he may have organic deviations, a reduced intellectual capacity, or sensory impairment, as long as his basic disorder does not impair his ability to make harmonious personal and social adaptations, he is usually regarded as emotionally sound or normal. It is necessary for him, then, to pass through the various development stages by *adapting* to both inner and outer stresses. Emotional disturbance, therefore, must be considered in terms of what the child's culture expects of him and what the people in his environment consider desirable. The age of the child and the normal stresses that may occur in each phase of development must be considered. For sound emotional development, a child needs good health and adequate intellectual development. He also needs parents who are relatively free from major emotional conflicts and a community which recognizes his value as a human being and encourages his participation in everyday activities. In addition, sound emotional development is dependent upon a minimum of traumatic incidents which the child must overcome if he is to be considered acceptable to society.

Most specialists concerned with emotional disturbance in children imply that childhood psychosis is a broad term which covers a number of problems. Two of these are of particular concern to the speech and hearing therapist: symbiotic psychosis and autism.

47   Symbiotic psychosis is described by Margaret S. Mahler in "On Child Psychosis and Schizophrenia," *Psychoanalytic Study of the Child,* VII (New York: International Universities Press, 1952), 286-305. Autism is discussed by Leo Kanner in "Early Infantile Autism," *Journal of Pediatrics,* XXV (1944), 211-17.

These two types of emotional disturbance are discussed in more detail later, but there are at least three other types of problems which should be mentioned here. One is called *irreversible ana-*

clitic depressions and occurs in some children who are hospitalized for long periods of time. Another is what some specialists refer to as childhood *schizophrenia,* where the child lives completely in a world of fantasy. Finally is the belief by many specialists that the brain-injured child, as described on pages 107–9 of this text, represents a specific type of childhood psychosis.

48   For more information concerning irreversible anaclitic depressions, read R. A. Spitz, "Hospitalism—a Follow-up Report," and "Hospitalism: An Inquiry into the Genesis of Psychiatric Conditions in Early Childhood," in *The Psychoanalytic Study of the Child,* I and II (New York: International Universities Press, 1945, 1946); Clemens Benda discusses the brain-injured child with reference to psychosis in *Developmental Disorders of Mentation and Cerebral Palsies* (New York: Grune & Stratton, Inc., 1952). See Lauretta Bender, *Psychopathology of Children with Organic Brain Disorders* (Springfield, Ill.: Charles C. Thomas, Publisher, 1956), for a discussion of schizophrenia in childhood.

Generally speaking, children with emotional disturbance can be differentiated from children whose delayed speech and language development reflect other etiology, primarily by the way they relate to other people. For example, the mentally retarded child may be delayed in speech acquisition and motor skills; he may have signs of physical stigmata, or congenital deformities associated with mental subnormality; and yet, as compared with the emotionally disturbed child, he always relates to people quickly, obviously, and usually warmly. The child with a hearing loss is also delayed in the acquisition of speech; he may have a motor problem due to vestibular or central involvement; and he may be able to respond to sound only when the intensity level supersedes his sensory deficit. But he is usually a friendly child and makes a definite, and usually lasting, identification with people around him. However, when a child is delayed in speech and language development and emotional disturbance is suspected as the causal factor, there are certain behavioral responses which are glaring deviations from the normal and which call for psychiatric evaluation. Some children appear to

49   Students concerned with emotional problems of children, particularly as they relate to speech development, should read J. T. Morrow's "A Psychiatrist Looks at the Non-Verbal Child," in *Exceptional Children* (April 1959), pp. 347-51. For a broad treatment of emotional problems in children, see J. L. Despert, *Emotional Problems in Children* (Utica: State Hospital Press, 1938).

be severely depressed, and they may demonstrate this depression by attempting partial self-destruction, as seen in head banging, self-hitting, or continual picking at open sores. Such self-destructive behavior strongly indicates their need for psychiatric evaluation. The child who lacks inhibitions to such a degree that he is assaultive or dangerous to others should also be seen for psychiatric appraisal. When delinquent behavior continues and does not alter despite modifications in the environment or attempts to help the child, the possibility of emotional disturbance should be considered. When a physically handicapped child does not respond within a reasonable amount of time to the procedures designed to alleviate or help him overcome his handicap, he, too, should be seen for psychiatric evaluation. The child with a learning problem which is not improved by usually effective re-educational techniques; the child with a speech problem who does not respond readily to usually successful retraining procedures; the child who in the absence of discernible physical cause for illness continues to complain; the child with a history of bizarre behavior, whether or not it is related to physical or intellectual handicaps; or a child showing withdrawal symptoms expressed by phobias and generally poor emotional tone or apathy should be referred for psychiatric evaluation in order to determine whether this is a primary or secondary cause of his inability.

50   For a case study of an emotionally disturbed child, see pages 120-22 of text, and for other case studies of various types of emotional disturbance, see The Psychoanalytic Study of the Child, IX (New York: International Universities Press, Inc., 1956).

HEARING LOSS

The relationship between speech and language development and well-functioning sensory modalities should be fairly obvious. In order to develop speech and language normally, we depend upon audition, which is our major source of incoming speech stimuli. We continue throughout life to use hearing for the purposes of monitoring or improving our communication. When hearing loss is present, its early detection is crucial to the child's total development, for the child must learn early in life to compensate for his loss by using other sensory modalities such as sight and touch.

Hearing loss, like other causes of delayed speech and language development, lies along a continuum representing various degrees of impairment. Deafness lies at one end of the continuum; minimal hearing loss, at the other. In between are various degrees of hearing loss. When a child is classified as *deaf*, it means that his ability to hear is not functional for the ordinary purposes for which hearing is used. Children who are born deaf are classified as *congenitally deaf*, and those who are born with normal hearing, but who later, through illness or accident, lose this function, are classified as *adventitiously deaf*. A hard-of-hearing child is one who has some degree of usable hearing, and, although his hearing is defective, he may be able to compensate for this loss to some degree. This compensation may be obtained through the use of a wearable hearing aid, which amplifies sound so that he can use his residual hearing effectively, and through auditory training, an educational procedure necessary for all children with hearing loss.

51 Read S. Richard Silverman's two chapters: "Clinical and Educational Procedures for the Deaf" and "Clinical and Educational Procedures for the Hard of Hearing," in *Handbook of Speech Pathology,* I. F. Travis, ed. (New York: Appleton-Century-Crofts, Inc., 1957), pp. 389-425.

If, and when, a child with a hearing loss develops speech, he usually has an abnormal vocal quality that may be staccato in sound or monotone. He may also have an articulation disorder, for his speech is mechanically faulty. Usually, the primary complaint of parents of a young child with hearing loss is that he does not respond to sound in his environment or that he does not appear to understand things said to him. Both of these behavioral responses are realistic. From a practical standpoint, a child who has a severe hearing loss will probably never have completely normal speech — a fact responsible for considerable anxiety on the part of parents and understandable frustration on the part of the child. It is not uncommon, therefore, for children with hearing loss frequently to have emotional problems which must be considered as adjuncts to their primary problem. Usually, when a young child is found to have a hearing loss, his social play is limited by his parents. They fear that he may be seriously hurt, or perhaps even killed, in general activities which require the identification of danger through the sense of hearing. Therefore, much of the usual childhood activities of a child with a hearing loss, particularly when the hearing loss is severe, is controlled to such an extent that his language experiences are limited.

> 52   For a further discussion of these topics, see the companion texts in the Prentice-Hall Foundations of Speech Pathology Series, *The Deaf*, by Louis Di Carlo, and *The Hard of Hearing*, by John J. O'Neill.

During the past 10 years, considerable strides have been taken in eliminating or reducing causal factors which contribute to *conductive* hearing loss. Such diseases as mastoiditis and other disorders of the middle ear which formerly contributed to middle-ear deafness, are now controlled to a large extent by drugs and early medical care. Therefore, the children we see now in clinical settings, such as nurseries for children with hearing impairment, or those children for whom we are attempting to ascertain the cause of delayed speech and language development, most frequently are found to have central rather than peripheral hearing impairments. In other words, most of the children we see for examination today, particularly where the focal point of the clinical evaluation is whether or not a hearing loss exists, have the type of hearing loss associated with dysfunction of the central nervous system rather than with problems of the middle ear. Hence, new detection methods, some of which have been designed recently, plus considerable time and clinical know-how, are needed in the differential diagnosis of hearing loss in young children.

> 53   One of the most complete treatments of this subject is H. R. Myklebust's *Auditory Disorders in Children: A Manual for Differential Diagnosis* (New York: Grune & Stratton, Inc., 1954), p. 377.

Obviously, early detection of these losses is extremely important to a child, in terms of speech and language development. Also, some of the therapeutic and teaching procedures found successful in helping children with middle-ear losses may not be applicable to children with central auditory disorders.

> 54   For additional information concerning a child with a peripheral hearing loss, read the description presented later in this text on pages 119-20. Additional case reports which differentiate the child with peripheral loss from one with central impairment can be found in Myklebust's *Auditory Disorders in Children* and McGinnis's *Aphasic Children*.

SPEECH DEPRIVATION AND IMMATURITY

The causes of delayed speech and language development discussed previously were concerned primarily with subnormal intelligence, sensory disabilities, central nervous system impairment, and emotional disturbance. In addition to these, delayed speech and language development can be caused by environmental deprivation. In order for the child to develop language and be able to express ideas orally, the environment in which the child lives must contain adequate speech stimulation. There have been cases reported of children who have been left alone most of the day during the critical periods of development and who, as the result of lack of attention and lack of stimulation, were significantly delayed in speech and language development.

55 A major contributor to information along these dimensions is R. A. Spitz. Read "Hospitalism: An Inquiry into the Genesis of Psychiatric Conditions in Early Childhood," in *Psychoanalytic Study of the Child* (New York: International Universities Press, 1945), pp. 53-74.

Conversely, it is possible also that a child may not develop speech and language if he is overprotected. This occurs sometimes in families where a child is the youngest of a number of children and the older siblings, as well as the parents, speak for him. Both lack of stimulation and overprotection have been known to cause delayed speech and language development.

56 Do a library search to locate descriptions of any of the following children who suffered communicative deprivation: 1. Kaspar Hauser; 2. Victor, the Wild Boy of Aveyrn; 3. Kamala, The Wolf Girl of India; 4. Lucas, the Baboon Boy of Africa; or 5. Tamosha of Salvador.

Some children with delayed speech and language development are generally immature, yet they give no evidence of obvious organic involvement. Early detection of speech and language problems is, of course, one of our major goals. However, in our concern for early detection of problems, we must avoid classifying a child as having a speech or hearing problem when actually such a problem does not exist. The so-called "immature" child, for example, may be seen for speech examination during a time when speech sounds are emerging or when he is mastering certain fine motor skills. Usually, during this period of development, his oral responses may not be valid indicators of his potential speech competency. Hence, care must be taken lest our emphasis on the need for early detection result in premature, inaccurate labeling.

When the cause of delayed speech and language development is immaturity, there will be times when we cannot determine how soon a child will develop adequate speech patterns. Counsel with parents might suggest that the child needs more time, that we must "wait and see." However, if we do suggest to parents that we must "wait and see," we should, at least, have some idea of how long the waiting period may be and, after waiting, we should know what it is we expect to see. If we make these demands on ourselves as we evaluate the speech development of an "immature" child, the risk involved in using the term *immaturity* as a waste-basket classification is reduced considerably. More important, we reduce the possibilities of unnecessarily classifying a child as having a problem — which could create inappropriate concern on the part of the parents and, perhaps, apprehension or confusion on the part of the child.

The term *immaturity* indicates the possibility of eventual maturity. Hence, in speech and language development, as in all other areas of development, these children would be expected to function, eventually, at a normal or near-normal level. Usually, these children develop speech more easily and perhaps more quickly in group-oriented programs. For this reason, they are often referred to nursery schools, kindergartens, or regular classrooms where natural stimulation procedures frequently result in equal, if not greater, gains in speech and language development than professionally planned programs.

57   This is discussed further by N. E. Wood in "Educational Evaluation of School Aged Children with Language Disorders," in W. Daley, *Speech and Language Therapy with the Brain Injured Child* (Washington, D. C.: The Catholic University of America Press, 1962).

In summary, the determination of causal factors in children with delayed speech and language development is a complex process. In our attempt to ascertain the causal factors of delayed speech and language development, it is well to keep several points in mind.

First, if a child has a severe delay in speech production, and if his language development is limited or disturbed, no one clinical index or clinical orientation can adequately classify the causal factors of the problem. Delayed speech and language development is a multiple problem and requires a multidiscipline approach.

Second, single tests usable for young children are not discriminating enough at the present time to differentiate causal factors when severe delay in speech development is present. Consideration of a child's individual problem, through the combined clinical judgments of specialists from various disciplines, probably will produce the best results.

Third, a coordinated approach, encompassing all known facets of the child's development, should be undertaken if the causal factors are to be differentiated. The point should be made, again, that speech and language development does not occur as an isolated function but rather as a continuous developmental process entailing the intellectual, motor, social, emotional, and sensory spheres.

Finally, a need for identifying causal factors is an inherent part of the need to determine the educational objectives for the child with delayed speech and language development. Only through an effort to identify the cause of the delayed speech and language development can the problem be interpreted satisfactorily to his parents and others concerned with his welfare. ᘓᘓᘓ

EVALUATIONS OF CHILDREN WITH DELAYED SPEECH AND LANGUAGE development are difficult to discuss in any precise manner, for the procedures can differ from examiner to examiner and from child to child. However, regardless of the techniques used or the test items selected, the evaluation usually proceeds through a series of steps not unlike those which are taken in any diagnostic procedure. Speech and language evaluations might be said to have three major procedural intentions: to clarify what it is we are attempting to evaluate; to accumulate information pertinent to the focal point of the evaluation; and to select the most effective way to solve the problem.

Why is it important to clarify the purpose of the examination? Primarily, so that the attention of the examining staff can be

3 *evaluation of children with delayed speech and language development*

directed toward the specific problem which must be solved. The evaluation takes on considerably more direction and significance when, at the outset, the intention of the examination is clear to all concerned. Probably it is safe to say that each child examined may require a slightly different evaluation approach, and that, therefore, the evaluation procedures must be tailored to those individual needs.

58 J. A. Carrell and J. L. Bangs have discussed the symptomatology, etiology, differential diagnosis, and treatment of delayed speech and language development in "Disorders of Speech Comprehension Associated with Idiopathic Language Retardation," *The Nervous Child*, IX (January 1951), No. 1, 64-76.

Why should the evaluation process be designed to accumulate information which is related specifically to the problem which must be solved? This may appear to be such an obvious point that it does not need to be questioned here. Nevertheless, this is where examinations frequently go awry, for it is at this stage of the examination that facts may be emphasized which *do not* pertain to the particular problem being studied, or important informational items, which *are* pertinent, may be overlooked or neglected. It might be interesting to note, for example, precisely how a child may perform on a detailed series of tests in all the motor, sensory, and intellectual spheres. However, if the main concern of the specific evaluation is to determine the child's readiness for therapy, for example, it may be more effective to explore the social and emotional development of the child initially, leaving the more intricate and involved testing to a later date, after the child has had an opportunity to adjust to a clinical atmosphere or to a therapeutic setting.

59   For a discussion of observation classes for children with delayed language, see Tina Bangs, "Evaluating Children with Language Delay," *Journal of Speech and Hearing Disorders*, XXVI (February 1961), 6-18. Contained in this article, also, are charts for recording observation of behavior and language development.

Why must care be exercised in the evaluation and sorting of the possible alternative solutions to the problem? It is at this point that the clinical process becomes an art as well as a science, for there is seldom only one solution to any clinical problem. Hence, as several alternatives become evident, during the examination, numerous questions may be raised by the examining staff: Should we work with the parents instead of the child? Should we schedule the child for an observational period of therapy with additional testing following the sessions? Would he benefit more from group or individual therapy? Does his problem present such a complex picture that additional testing is needed before final decisions can be made? Is this problem one which requires more time for maturation before any professional intervention should be recommended? Should the child be referred to some other program in the community rather than the one with which we are associated? These are examples of the types of questions which staff members may ask, and they represent some of the different kinds of alternatives which may result from the examination sequence. Therefore, as we evaluate these possible alternatives in terms of the possible results of each, we may find that one alternative, or perhaps a combination of several, represents the best clinical solution to the problem we have been asked to consider.

60   This concept is explored in more detail in W. G. Hardy, "Problems of
Audition, Perception, and Understanding," *The Volta Review*, LVIII
(September 1956), No. 7, 300.

How much time is required to sort these various alternatives so that an appropriate clinical decision might be reached? At times, the parents of children with delayed speech and language development, as well as the specialists who referred these children for examination, fail to recognize the large amounts of time which may be required to administer the tests, interpret the results, and prepare the examination reports, all of which are necessary parts of the examination. Because of this unawareness, parents and specialists alike may become impatient for answers to their questions or anxious about the results of the examination. In order to reduce these reactions to some degree, it would seem wise for the examiner to estimate the amount of time entailed in those time-consuming activities which are necessary but which frequently may not be recognized as part of the examination procedures.

These activities, as well as the time required to carry them out, can vary with the purpose of the examination. For example, suppose that the purpose of the examination is to provide parental guidance and counsel rather than further observation or therapy for the child. Then, in addition to the time required for the examination procedures, additional time will be needed for conferences with the parents in order to help them understand their child's needs more completely and to provide them with suggestions for managing their child at home.

By the same token, if the purpose of the examination is to evaluate the child's speech and language development in terms of a broader, more comprehensive disorder (for example, cerebral palsy or mental retardation), then the results of the speech and language evaluation must be integrated and related to the results of other tests which have been completed or scheduled. Only in this way can the child's over-all probem be assessed and his total needs be evaluated. Again, in addition to the examination procedures, the necessary staff discussions and report writing will require additional staff time.

On occasion, a child is referred for a speech and language evaluation with the specific request that a report of the findings be forwarded to the referral source prior to any interpretation of the test results to the child's parents. Requests such as these are made, usually, to avoid the possible confusion which might result from the isolated interpretations of results by different specialists each representing a different specialty. In such instances, the referring specialist may ask specific questions about the current status of the child's speech and language development, or he may request a professional opinion as to the potential communication abilities of the child. In order to provide lucid and comprehensive answers to these questions, considerable time and care are necessary for preparing the report in such a way that an accurate interpretation of findings is assured and any misunderstanding of test results avoided.

In some instances, the examination requires a differential diagnosis of the numerous causes of delayed speech and language development. In an examination such as this, the focus must be a broad one, and it usually requires separate examinations of the child's vision, audition, intelligence, and emotional stability, as well as an evaluation of his capacity to learn or his ability to use linguistic symbols. Prior to the interpretation of the results of all of these separate tests, the findings must be integrated to form a composite clinical picture. A large segment of time may be required, therefore, to review the findings of the separate reports, and several staff meetings may be necessary to coordinate the various opinions.

61   For a detailed discussion of procedures in diagnosis and appraisal, read
      W. Johnson, F. Darley, and Spriestersbach, *Diagnostic Methods in
      Speech Pathology* (New York: Harper & Row, Publishers, 1963).

Sufficient time, alone, obviously cannot guarantee competent evaluations, because the adequacy of the test procedures, the accuracy of the interpretation, and the comprehensiveness of the report are all related directly to the competency of the examiner. This competence, which grows with professional preparation and experience, reflects more than knowledge of speech and language development. It reflects the examiner's thoughtful speculations about the intention of the examination sequence, the limitations of the individual tests, the demands of the interpretation of findings, and the responsibility inherent in the resulting recommendations. All of these points emphasize one fact clearly: no clinician becomes a good one only by reading books, or by taking courses, or by testing children. Rather, it is the combination of all these factors, plus that special something — call it talent, call it a gift, call it the ability to relate empathically — which makes the difference between a "mediocre technician" and a "superior clinician."

In general, information about a child's communication problem is obtained from three sources: the history of the problem, observations of behavior, and evaluations of the child's responses on specific tasks or in specific test situations. It cannot be stressed too strongly that, although each of these sources of information is important separately, effective and accurate clinical evaluations require that all available information about the specific problem being studied should be integrated to form a logical unit before final clinical decisions can be made.

HISTORY TAKING

Most examinations of children with delayed speech and language development begin with an accumulation of information about the child's past and present status. Usually, this information is reported by the child's parents, his guardian, or someone immediately responsible for his welfare. The initial interview is of major importance to the total evaluation of the child on several counts.

First, it is important that the information obtained at the initial interview be accurate and comprehensive. Because of the need for accuracy and thoroughness, the interviewer must be skilled in asking questions in such a way that the informant understands what types of answers are expected from him and so that cooperation between the interviewer and the informant is assured.

Second, we must recognize that the effect which the initial interviewer has on the informant frequently is perpetuated throughout subsequent testing. Since the initial interview is usually the first contact made with the informant, the effects of this session often are lasting ones. If the interviewer is unable to elicit the cooperation and confidence of the informant at this session, it is possible that this lack of cooperation and this lack of confidence may continue throughout the total examination process.

Third, in order to interpret the reported information adequately, the interviewer must have a comprehensive knowledge of speech and language development and the numerous possible causes of delayed speech and language development. There is little question that information obtained without purpose is a waste of time for both the informant and the interviewer. Further, all information that is reported is not of equal importance to the problem being studied. It is the selection of pertinent facts meaningful to the problem being studied which represents the real challenge.

This challenge is heightened by the fact that the history of the child's speech and language usually is reported by his parents. Therefore, a certain amount of bias in the information obtained must be expected. Frequently parents can describe their child's general behavior at home with adequate objectivity, but the parents are rare who can estimate objectively the more crucial aspects of their child's behavior. Generally speaking, parents cannot be relied upon to present a coherent or valid picture of the child's perform ance in areas such as social competence, mental abilities, and motor skills.

62   For an interesting treatment of history-taking, particularly the question of whether or not the child should be present when questions about his problems are being asked, see Chapter 28, "History-Taking," in Bakwin and Bakwin, *Clinical Management of Behavior Disorders in Children* (Philadelphia: W. B. Saunders Co., 1960), pp. 229-33.

The methods used to obtain case history information vary. Some interviewers ask literally hundreds of questions, such as: How would you describe the environmental climate into which this child was born? Were there any complications in the birth process? Has the child had any diseases, particularly those accompanied by high temperature? What are the attitudes of others in the family, particularly siblings, toward this child? What were the results of previous examinations? How would you describe the child's behavior at home; in group play; on shopping trips? Other examiners prefer a nondirective approach and ask the informant simply to "Tell me about the problem," with little or no guidance or specific questions from the examiner. Regardless of the method used, the important thing about history taking is to determine *why* the information is being obtained, *how* it will be used, and *to what extent* the questions and resulting answers are pertinent to the total examination.

The atmosphere surrounding the history-taking procedure is extremely important. It is not enough for the examiner to assure the informant that all information obtained will remain confidential, or that the questions are not being asked because of the examiner's insatiable curiosity. The informant must be made to feel that these questions are important, pertinent, and relative to the total examination procedures. Every effort should be made to put the informant at ease. For example, the room where the interview is held should be removed from other clinical activities so that confidentiality of information may be ensured, and the informant should not be pressured to give information which he is not ready to discuss. One of the major mistakes that a beginning interviewer frequently makes is to attempt to obtain all of the information he considers necessary during the first interview session. This is seldom a successful approach. Frequently not one but perhaps a series of interviews needs to be scheduled, giving the informant an opportunity to understand more fully the kinds of information the examiner needs to know. We must provide that necessary period of time during which rapport and trust can develop between informant and examiner. In nearly all cases, a series of interview sessions permits a more relaxed climate for obtaining information, particularly information which is extremely personal.

Whether a direct method of interviewing is used (where specific questions are asked, in an attempt to get specific kinds of information), or whether the interviewer uses an indirect approach (where general questions are asked and information is recorded as presented and reorganized later in terms of specific areas of clinical interest), there are some general broad areas of the history which should be covered. These areas include information pertaining to the prenatal, birth, and postnatal history; the informant's estimates of the child's social, emotional, motor, and mental abilities; and, of course, specific information about the child's speech and language development.

63   For a more complete discussion of the case history and for suggestions
     pertaining to the various methods used for obtaining case history data,
     the student is urged to study the detailed and comprehensive treatment
     of these procedures in *Diagnostic Methods in Speech Pathology* by
     three outstanding clinicians, W. Johnson, F. Darley, and D. C. Spriesters-
     bach (New York: Harper & Row, Publishers, 1963).

Identifying Information

It may seem absurd to emphasize the importance of obtaining and recording accurate identifying information in a case history. But, as most supervisors of speech and hearing services know, case histories frequently do not contain adequate identifying information for efficient case history storage or retrieval. Obtaining identifying information — the name of the child, his address, the date of his birth; the father's and mother's names, ages, and occupations; the siblings by age and sex; the referral source; the family physician's name and address; the last known date when the child was examined by his family doctor or pediatrician — serves a dual purpose. First, because most of the information of this type is factual and can be obtained without difficulty at the initial interview, it provides the informant with an opportunity to form a clinical bond with the examiner prior to discussing more personal information. Second, it provides the examiner with an opportunity to estimate the informant's level of intelligence and emotional stability, and so enables him to phrase his questions in such a way as to obtain the most valid information possible.

64 For further information on this point, consult Frederic Darley's text, *Diagnosis and Appraisal of Communication Disorders* in the Prentice-Hall Foundations of Speech Pathology Series.

Prenatal History

Generally speaking, the prenatal history of any child may be difficult to obtain and, if it is provided by the mother, the validity of the information may be questionable. Few mothers can report, with accuracy, information about the prenatal life of a child, particularly if the child is one of several. In essence, the aim of obtaining prenatal history information is to determine, inasmuch as possible, whether there were any unusual conditions surrounding the prenatal life of a child. However, it is important to note that some children with unremarkable histories may have severe problems in communication and other problems whereas other children with severely abnormal prenatal, natal, and postnatal histories may have few or no complications. If speech and language development is severely delayed, an attempt usually is made to obtain information about the mother's health during pregnancy. A history of miscarriages, hemorrhages, or spotting can suggest that the onset of the problem might have occurred during the prenatal period. Rh incompatibility, toxemia, the mother's use of medication during the prenatal period, and the mother's need for X ray or surgery during the prenatal period have been causally related to organic problems. Anemia, extreme nausea, severe depression, fatigue, emotional upset, and hypertension also may be contributing factors to a prenatal problem.

65   For a more detailed discussion of these terms, the student should refer
      to the texts noted previously: *Clinical Management of Behavior Dis-*
      orders in Children and *Diagnostic Methods in Speech Pathology.* Also
      see "Differential Diagnosis of Communication Disorders in Children Re-
      ferred for Hearing Tests," in *AMA Archives,* LX (October 1954), 468-77,
      written by S. Kastein and E. P. Fowler, Jr.

Accurate information about the prenatal life of a child can be obtained only from medical records. However, these records are not easily available, particularly to nonmedical personnel. Frequently, when these records are available, it is found that the information which might be pertinent to a communication disorder has not been recorded, unless the problem was recognized as a vital or unusual complicating factor.

Birth History

A complete and accurate birth history also is difficult to obtain, and, again, is an area which may not provide objective or valid information when obtained only through parental reports. The obstetrical report may be available to the family physician, but unless some particular problem occurred during the birth process, the report usually will be negative. Mothers do remember with fair accuracy what occurred during the birth process and other conditions which may be present at the time of birth, if these facts were in any way remarkable. But the presence of factors such as jaundice, prematurity, abnormal presentation, prolonged labor, anoxia, and placenta previa requires identification by a physician before they can be considered possible contributing factors to organic problems.

Postnatal History

Although both the prenatal and birth history information are difficult to obtain, and when obtained from parental reports are highly suspect, the information obtained from parents concerning the postnatal history of the child usually is more valid and more reliable. Mothers usually can report if they noticed any scars, deformations, or bruises when they first saw the child following birth. They usually can report the child's general health and well-being accurately, and they usually know whether or not the child had seizures or other complications during his early life. Information concerning childhood diseases usually is fairly accurate, particularly concerning familiar or fairly easily identified childhood illnesses such as measles, chicken pox, whooping cough, diphtheria, scarlet fever, mumps, and influenza. If at all possible, it is important to ascertain which of these illnesses were associated with high temperatures and how long these temperatures were sustained. Of particular importance is a report of diseases, such as meningitis or encephalitis, which are associated with disorders of the central nervous system. Any diseases affecting the middle ear, such as tonsillitis, sinusitis, otitis media, and nasal allergy, should be noted, and any unusual episodes in the child's life, such as accidents or emotional traumas, should be explored, as should any other unusual condition surrounding the prenatal, birth, or postnatal history of the child.

66   Additional attention to history information can be found in R. L. Clemmens, "Minimal Brain Damage in Children," *Children*, VIII (1962), 179-83.

Information about the history of a child's problem will, of course, vary with the suspected cause of the problem. Regardless of the cause, however, the various developmental stages should be explored. If a child is delayed in sitting alone, walking alone, talking in words, talking in sentences, bladder training, feeding, or dressing himself, the reason for the delay should be investigated.

Speech and hearing clinics usually develop their own examination forms, including specific lists of history questions pertaining to delayed speech and language development. Knowing which questions to ask is of major importance, of course, but even more important is knowing what to do with the information once it has been obtained.

67   For a sample chart used to record the case history of speech and hearing disorders, see C. Van Riper, *Speech Correction: Principles and Methods*, 4th Ed. (Englewood Cliffs, N. J.: Prentice-Hall, Inc., 1963), particularly Appendix D, "The Case History," pp. 491-502. For an informative discussion of history interpretation, see Chapter 5 in H. R. Myklebust, *Auditory Disorders in Children* (New York: Grune & Stratton, Inc., 1954).

In summary, the information concerning the prenatal, birth, and postnatal histories is best obtained from hospital records. But hospital records are not easily available and, if available, not always complete. In addition, parents have considerable difficulty remembering specific items concerning one child if there are several children in the family. Even parents of an only child may not be able to report information accurately or completely. It remains part of the clinical judgment of the examiner to know how far information of this sort should be pursued. Again, it is well to remember that the importance of history taking is related directly to three basic points: *why* the information is being obtained; *how* the history information will be used in the total examination; *to what degree* the answers to questions should be pursued before final clinical decisions can be made.

OBSERVATION OF BEHAVIOR

One of the most productive sources of information about a child with delayed speech and language development is the observation of his behavior in both structured and unstructured situations. Hence, observations of a child's behavior before, during, and after the examination sequence may pay clinical dividends. Because of the important role that the observation of behavior plays in the evaluation, it is regrettable that so little is done to prepare the beginning student to know *what* and *how* to observe. It is unfortunate that observational procedures receive so little academic attention from those responsible for the professional preparation of speech and hearing therapists. Too often it is taken for granted that these students, who are in the process of being academically trained in a specialty, know how to observe instinctively. However, there is a distinct difference between "observing" a child's behavior and "looking at" a child.

The term *observation* implies a dynamic evaluation of responses and requires that the observer make every effort to understand the implications of the behavioral interactions which are observed. Observation is not a passive, undirected, or unlearned process: If inferences about the behavior of a child are to be drawn from observations, then observation procedures must be as scientific as possible. It is not enough for us to record descriptively that a child behaved in a particular way. We must attempt to ascertain *why* and *when* he behaved in this manner, and *to what extent* his behavior deviated from what normally would be expected in the situation being observed.

Clues as to *what* to observe can often be found in the report of the child's behavior at home. Parents may report that their child is a head-banger, a body-rocker, a thumb-sucker, that he has severe and uncontrollable temper tantrums, that he mouths objects, or that he eats nonedibles. They may report that he harmfully attacks himself or others, that he masturbates, that he seems unaware of danger, that there is severe sibling rivalry in the home, that he is a bed-wetter, that he is destructive, and that he is either aggressive or withdrawn. They may add that he has a feeding problem or a sleeping problem, that he has a short attention span, and that he is difficult, if not impossible, to manage in the home environment. Yet, although this may be a valid report of the child's behavior at home, the child may give no evidence of these kinds of behavioral deviations when observed in a clinical setting. The opposite may also occur. The child who is reported as having no remarkable behavioral deviations in the home situation may in a strange clinical environment be extremely difficult to manage. More typically, if the parents report extremely deviant behavior in the home environment, similar behavior also will be noted in the clinical setting. In cases such as these, it is important not only to note how the child behaves in various situations, but also to decide what his behavior may mean in terms of the total examination sequence.

Suppose, however, that there are no parental reports available, or none which indicate gross behavioral deviations. Or, as frequently occurs, suppose that the observer has not had access to the case history prior to observing the child. How, then, can the observer record what he observes so that his report will be meaningful? Although the abilities of the observer become more accurate and more thorough with increased experience and professional knowledge, the beginning student must devise some system for recording his observations in a logical sequence. Frequently, a chronologic record serves this purpose, beginning with the first time the child is seen and through a series of observations until the examination is completed.

Our first encounter with the child usually is in the waiting room, prior to the examination. Here we have an opportunity to observe him without his knowledge — a situation which may give us some insight into the way in which he relates to his parents or others. Equally important, it provides us with an opportunity to observe the way in which his parents and others relate to him.

Whether or not he will be cooperative during the subsequent examination procedures can be determined, to a large extent, by the way in which he arrives at the examination room. Was he pushed, led, dragged, chased, carried, or accompanied? Was he able to separate from his mother, father, guardian, relative, nurse, next-door neighbor, or whoever else brought him for examination? If the examiner preferred to examine the child without others in the room, was the child able to accompany the examiner alone and without undue disturbance?

How did the child behave as he entered the examination room? Was he curious, shy, anxious, hesitant, eager, unaware of his surroundings, fearful, unconcerned, interested? If there were toys in the examination room or other objects of interest to children, did he wait for an invitation to select one, or did he go directly to something that seemed to interest him? Did he wander around the room without attending to any one object, crawl under the furniture, sit down at the test table, wait for the examiner to tell him what to do, look around the room in some attempt to appraise his surroundings? If the mother and/or father were in the room with him, did he stay close to them, requiring that the examiner entice him, in some way, to cooperate? Did he insist on being close to his mother during the testing situation? Was his behavior on entering the test room appropriate for his age?

During the examination, did he cooperate with the examiner, or did he refuse to participate in any of the test activities? Was his attention span unusually short for his chronological age? Was he hyperactive to such an extent that the examiner had to bring him back to the test table time and time again? Did he demonstrate

68   See Earl A. Loomis, Jr., "Autistic and Symbiotic Syndromes in Children,"
      in N. E. Wood, *Language Development and Language Disorders: A
      Compendium of Lectures* (Society for Research in Child Development,
      Inc.), XXV (1960), No. 3, 41-48.

any of the unusual hand or finger play sometimes seen in emotionally disturbed children? Did he insist on continuing with one activity, refusing to participate in others to such an extent that his behavior could be considered perseverative? Did he appear to be clumsy, uncoordinated? Did he use echolalia? How did he make his wants known to the examiner? How did he respond to the examiner's request to participate in particular tasks? Did he have eye contact with the examiner? Did he make any vocal sounds that had an unusual quality? Did he use echolalia, random speech, gesture language?

How long could he maintain his attention to the testing situation? Was the examiner able to complete the test battery? If the parents were in the room during the testing, how did they respond to his successes or failures? What was his general physical appearance? Did he seem to be adequately developed in terms of height and weight? Did he have any obvious physical anomalies? Was he appropriately dressed, and did he appear to be well nurtured and cared for? Did he give any evidence of tics, drooling, nail biting, or tremors?

As he prepared to leave the room, did he seem pleased with his performance during the test situation? Had he established some type of relationship with the examiner? Did he show promise in his ability to benefit from therapy or treatment?

In essence, recorded observations should form a constellation or a clinical picture that either supports or negates information items reported in the case history and the results of specific tests. Although some behavioral deviations are expected in all children when they are in strange environments, it is the consistency with which deviate behavior occurs and the patterning of his over-all behavior which marks one child as having a behavior problem and not another. Further, it is the effect of a child's behavior on others in his environment as well as on himself, which indicates that his behavior problem requires professional attention. Hence, a young child of two or three who is shy and fearful and cannot be separated from his mother for test purposes might well be considered quite normal in his response to a strange situation. However, a child of six or seven who behaves in this manner, in the same clinical setting, may be considered grossly immature or even emotionally disturbed.

69   For suggestions on specific behavior requiring evaluation and how to record observations, see Tina Bangs, "Evaluating Children with Language Delay," *Journal of Speech and Hearing Disorders,* XXVI (February 1961), 5-18.

Observation of behavior is not an isolated clinical activity which can be evaluated apart from the history of the problem or the examination of the child. Observation serves as a network, tying together pertinent history items and responses to testing procedures. These components together form a clinical pattern which eventually points to a tentative diagnosis of the primary problem.

The ability to be a critical, objective observer is learned. It develops from both theoretical and clinical experience. For this reason it is difficult, perhaps impossible, to discuss observation, as an isolated process, without an opportunity to demonstrate those behavior patterns being discussed. Yet the value of observation cannot be overstated. Supervised observation is regarded as a testing ground for potential clinicians, for it is through the observation of experienced clinicians that the future capabilities of students in training are developed. It is important, therefore, that both beginning and advanced clinicians continue throughout the course of their professional activities to observe human behavior, particularly the responses of those individuals for whom they provide professional services.

Undoubtedly, observation reports should be a summation of *facts,* and, particularly in the case of beginning students, the possibility of reporting *as fact* behavior which actually did not occur is not unusual. Some of this inaccuracy may stem from reading the case history. After noting the behavior reported by parents and the interviewer, the student may believe that he has observed certain behavior patterns simply because these responses were reported previously. Therefore, the beginning student must be cautioned to report actually what did occur when he was acting as an observer, and to separate observation from inference.

At the same time, however, the student must learn to link these observations with known facts about the child's problem, and, the warning to "stick to the facts" should not serve to dampen his attempt to draw clinical conclusions from the behavior he has observed.

For example, the beginning student frequently finds himself in an observation room, separated from the examiner and child by a two-way-vision mirror. Sometimes he has little or no knowledge of the type of problem he has been scheduled to observe. Warned that observation must be coupled with facts, students have a tendency to write stereotyped kinds of observation reports, consisting frequently of terse descriptions of what they have seen in the examination room: "The child entered the room. The examiner took the child to the test table. The examiner showed the child a puzzle. The child attempted to put the puzzle together. He was not able to perform adequately on this task. The examiner selected another test which the child was able to do. After the testing was completed, the examiner took the child from the room." Obviously, this type of observation report, void of any personal thoughts and lacking in any future applicability, is worthless to both the observer and the clinician responsible for the observer's professional training.

In brief, the student must learn to submit his observations to crucial tests, checking what he has reported as "facts" against the final history report and test results, before he attempts to interpret the meaning of this behavior. In this way, his observations and clinical impressions of the child's behavior will be sharpened and his reports will be less vague and misleading, more accurate, and more complete.

The importance of clinical observation cannot be overstated and the need for professional training in this area cannot be overemphasized, for the opportunity provided students to observe clinical activities under the guidance of master teachers and diagnosticians is one of their most valuable learning situations. Only in this way can the theory learned in the classroom be combined with the observations of practical application. Supervised observation, then, provides the vital link between theory and clinical practice.

SPECIFIC AREAS OF TESTING

One of the primary responsibilities of a speech and hearing therapist is to know *how, when,* and *why* to refer a child for specific testing; another is to know enough about test procedures so that he can interpret the results of the examination accurately. The purpose of the discussion which follows is to consider the evaluation of speech and language development in terms of these responsibilities. It should be clear that it is not the aim of this discussion to recommend specific tests, nor to compare or contrast the validity or reliability ratings of currently available tests or scales. Rather, the intention here is to suggest some general concepts regarding speech and language evaluations, leaving the selection of specific tests, and the selection of methods used to explore specific areas, where they rightly belong — within the prerogative of the individual examiner.

70 For a summary of available tests, see the companion text of this series, *Diagnosis and Appraisal of Communication Disorders,* by Frederic Darley.

Usually, in a speech and language evaluation, an attempt is made to examine each aspect of behavior separately, determining how a child functions in terms of motor skills, mental abilities, auditory capacities, social maturity, emotional stability, and language development. However, even though we may evaluate these areas separately, we must keep in mind that when these specific aspects of behavior are observed in their natural states, they almost never are seen in isolation. In fact, to the contrary, they are always integrated and associated with each other.

Therefore, although our attention may be focused on the evaluation of motor skills, we cannot divorce these skills from related factors, such as *retention* of motor patterns, memory, and comprehension of the examiner's directions, all of which may influence the motor activity exhibited. Similarly, when we evaluate intelligence, we also are concerned with perception, reception, concept formation, and language development. This same type of broad relationship holds true in the evaluation of hearing, social maturity, emotional stability, and other behavioral aspects.

MOTOR SKILLS

The most immediate purpose of the evaluation of motor performance is, of course, to determine which motor skills can be performed without difficulty and which cannot. In the evaluation of delayed speech and language development, the speech and hearing specialist is concerned primarily with three broad areas of motor evaluation: *General Motor Function, Visual-Motor Function, and Speech-Motor Function.*

General Motor Function,

as it relates to speech and language development, can be evaluated from at least five separate standpoints: locomotor function, balance, cerebral dominance, manual dexterity, and psychomotor behavior.

Locomotor Function

Gross motor dysfunction is a major key to possible impairment of the central nervous system. Obvious motor dysfunctions, such as paralysis or paresis, can be noted without too much difficulty by watching the child walk around the room, or by observing his attempt to manipulate large objects. Less obvious locomotor problems may be noted when the examiner observes the child's gait, stance, speed of movement, or range of movement. The gait of the child, for example, should be freely moving without evidence of limping, toe-walking, stiffness, or the dragging of one foot. The normal stance of a child is usually considered to be approximately the width of his shoulders. While observing a child's stance it is possible also to observe his speed and range of movement and to note whether these movements are adequate for normal motor activity. One way to appraise the child's adequacy of movement is to decide whether or not the speed and range are appropriate to the activity being observed.

71   For further information about locomotor function and its evaluation, and the motor development of the young child, see Nancy Bayley, *The Development of Motor Abilities During the First Three Years* (published by the Society for Research in Child Development, 1935).

Balance

Problems in balance can suggest cerebellar ataxia, vestibular disorders, or other problems associated with organic impairment. At times, balance problems can be noted by watching the way in which a child moves around in his environment. Another way to observe the child's balance is to ask him to stand with feet together, eyes closed, and arms extended, while the examiner notes the degree of sway which is present (both forward and backward, and side to side). Severe problems in balance are strong indications that a child should be referred for medical examination.

72   Problems of balance may be linked also with auditory disorders, as well as with disorders stemming from central nervous system impairment without involvement of the sensory system. For a discussion of motor capacity and the examination of motor function, see H. R. Myklebust, *Auditory Disorders in Children* (New York: Grune & Stratton, Inc., 1954), pp. 307-13.

Cerebral Dominance

It has not been clearly shown from an anatomical or physiological standpoint how problems of cerebral dominance are related to delayed speech and language development, yet evidence of mixed laterality or contra-dominance is observed frequently in children with delayed speech and other language-learning problems. Because of this relationship, most speech and language evaluations include tests of laterality, particularly tests of handedness and footedness. These tests of laterality can be done rather simply, and they are easily recorded. In no instance should these tests be considered a substitute for a neurologic examination, but frequently they reveal information which may be useful to the speech and hearing therapist in selecting or carrying out therapeutic procedures.

In testing for handedness, the examiner might place a small object in front of the child between his left hand and his right hand. The child is asked to pick up the object and hand it to the examiner, who is sitting across from him. The examiner notes in three out of five trials whether the child prefers to use his right hand or his left hand in this type of activity. There are other occasions on which the examiner can observe which hand the child uses routinely, or if he has developed a preference, for throughout the entire examination sequence the preferred hand in manual tasks is noted.

Footedness can be observed by having the child kick a ball or some other small object which has been placed between his feet, directly in front of him. Notation of which foot he prefers to use is noted in three out of five trials.

Although eye preference is explored frequently by having a child sight through a tube or through a hole cut in a piece of paper, preferred eye use is not considered an aspect of cerebral dominance, because both eyes are used simultaneously in all normal visual activities. Nevertheless, if it is found that the child's eye preference is counter to his hand and foot preference, this contra-dominance may be a clue to subsequent reading disorders.

73 Information concerning laterality (the preferential use of one side) can be found in S. T. Orton, *Reading, Writing, and Speech Problems in Children* (New York: W. W. Norton & Company, Inc., 1935). This text has become a valuable resource for the speech and hearing therapist

and is useful in the detection of reading, writing, and speech problems in young children. For information concerning the use of laterality tests, read W. C. Barger, "An Experimental Approach to Aphasia and Non-Reading Children," *American Journal of Orthopsychiatry, XXIII (1953),* 158.

Manual Dexterity

Locomotor function, balance, and cerebral dominance represent large, unrefined, motor activities and, therefore, are referred to as *gross* motor functions. In contrast, some motor skills require *fine* motor coordination, as seen in tasks requiring manual dexterity. Tests of manual dexterity usually include an evaluation of a child's ability to grasp objects, to point accurately to previously selected directions, and to grip objects or things in an effective and useful manner. Fine motor skills can be evaluated by using paper-pencil tests. Some of these tasks require the tracing of mazes or the copying of geometric designs, letters, and numbers. Others use picture drawing, some of which are requested specifically by the examiner (draw-a-man, draw-a-tree, and so forth), or the child may be asked simply to "draw a picture." It is important to note, while observing these activities, that some children who have no obvious *gross* motor disability may be found to have difficulty with *fine* motor tasks.

74   In "A Comparison of Motor Skills of Mentally Retarded and Normal Children," in *Exceptional Children* (April 1959), pp. 352-54, Clifford E. Howe came to some interesting conclusions regarding the education of children with subnormal scores on a series of motor tasks. Do you think the implications drawn from this study could be applied advantageously to children with delayed speech and language development?

Psychomotor Behavior

Although some children are able to perform adequately on both gross and fine motor tasks, they may be unable to control certain motor responses. These psychomotor problems may include: *tremors* (slight, palsied-like movements of the hands or head), *overflow movements* (movements which go past the original intention of the activity, for example, reaching beyond an object, or to one side of it, when attempting to pick it up), *tics* (quick, involuntary movements of the muscles of the head or face, particularly the eyes and mouth), and *extraneous movements* (unnecessary tapping of fingers or feet, or any uncontrolled movement of the arms). All of these psychomotor problems have been seen in children with known central nervous system impairment. Tics and certain extraneous movements have been associated also with emotional problems.

Visual-Motor Function

Although some children may have adequate visual acuity and only a slight, generalized motor problem, their inability to function on tasks which require the integration of visual and motor functions often points to a problem of incoordination. There are various ways to observe this combined activity. For example, the use of form boards and paper-pencil tests provides an opportunity to observe visual-motor performance in a young child, and, in older children, writing activities can be used to evaluate visual-motor performances.

Form boards, standardized for various age levels, frequently are used to observe the way in which a child handles materials and to determine the time required for him to complete the required performance. Not only is it important to observe his successes or failures in completing the tasks, but the ways in which he attempts to complete the tests should be noted also. For example, trial-and-error placement usually is associated with mental retardation, whereas the need to line up the inserts before placing them has been associated with central nervous system impairment.

75 See Chapter III, "Perception and Perceptual Disturbances of Brain-Injured Children," in *Psychopathology and Education of the Brain-Injured Child*, by A. A. Strauss and L. E. Lehtinen (New York: Grune & Stratton, Inc., 1947), pp. 28-53.

Paper-pencil tasks may be used to observe the combined abilities of prehension, manual dexterity, and visual-motor integration. In these tasks, the child imitates the drawing of the examiner (for example, geometric designs: circles, squares, triangles, and so forth). Here, again, it is not only the success or failure with which he accomplishes this task that should be noted, but the way in which he attempts to reproduce the design.

76 *Draw a Man Test,* designed and studied by F. Goodenough, was based upon this principle and has been used as a test of intelligence with

considerable success. However, before drawings can be used as intelligence tests, considerable professional training is required in the administration of the test and in the interpretation of test results.

Speech-Motor Function

Evaluation of the speech-motor system includes an oral cavity examination, with special emphasis on the movement of the articulators; an articulation test in which defective sounds can be noted;
and a description of the voice, particularly the ability or inability
to sustain tone.

Examination of the oral cavity includes a report of any deviations
of the lips, teeth, palate, jaws, or tongue. The ease and rhythm
of the lateral or forward movements of the tongue and the ability
to lift the tongue on both a voluntary and involuntary basis are
also recorded. The way in which the tongue, teeth, and jaws function as articulators is an important focal point of this examination,
and any indication of dysarthria or apraxia should be noted.

77   For additional information about dysarthria, see the article by W. G.
      Peacher, "The Etiology and Differential Diagnosis of Dysarthria," in
      Journal of Speech and Hearing Disorders, XV (1950), 252-65; and
      Dysarthric Speech, by E. Froeschels (Magnolia, Mass.: Expression Co.,
      1952). Information about apraxia can be found in *Agnosia, Apraxia,
      Aphasia,* by J. M. Nielsen (New York: Paul B. Hoeber, Inc., 1948).

If the child has some speech, the use of standard articulation
tests supplies the examiner with a comprehensive picture of which
sounds are defective and in which positions (initial, medial, or
final) these defective sounds occur. The degree of impairment is
determined by established speech development schedules.

78   See W. Johnson, F. Darley, and D. Spriestersbach, *Diagnostic Methods
      in Speech Pathology* (New York: Harper & Row, Publishers, 1963),
      pp. 80-110, for normative data in articulation development.

Evidence of jargon, echolalia, substitution, omission, or distor-
tion of specific sounds should be reported, as well as whether or
not the child can imitate sounds accurately. Because some children
use speech in some situations and not others, these occasions, and
the type of speech used, should be noted. Detailed discussions of
speech evaluations can be found in several texts.

79   Robert Milisen, "Methods of Evaluation and Diagnosis of Speech Disorders," in *Handbook of Speech Pathology,* L. E. Travis, ed. (New York: Appleton-Century-Crofts, Inc., 1957), pp. 264, 309; Charles Van Riper, *Speech Correction: Principles and Methods,* 4th Ed. (Englewood Cliffs, N. J.: Prentice-Hall, Inc., 1963), p. 528; Wendell Johnson, Frederic Darley, and D. C. Spriestersbach, *Diagnostic Methods in Speech Pathology* (New York: Harper & Row, Publishers, 1963), p. 347.

Also, as can be seen in those references mentioned above, the ability of the child to vary the pitch of his voice, and also its volume, rate, and rhythm, can be extremely important clues in the differentiation of causal factors for delayed speech and language development. The voice of a child with hearing loss usually is stereotyped, reflecting his inability to hear pitch variations; a child with a severe emotional problem may merely vocalize in a staccato rhythm, with extreme variations in volume, because this is the way he can best express himself; a mentally retarded child may have a flat, expressionless voice because his entire means of communication are limited.

80   For additional information concerning voice differences, read Levin's *Voice and Speech Disorders: Medical Aspects* (Springfield, Ill.: Charles C. Thomas, Publisher, 1962).

The evaluation of a child's general motor function, visual-motor function, and speech-motor function can provide many clues which are useful, but if the motor evaluation is to have any real significance to the total speech and language evaluation, then motor skills must be evaluated in terms of their effect upon the child's ability to communicate. Obviously, the relationship between motor skills and speech and language development is not revealed by indicating how many times a child can hop on one foot, or how many objects he can catch without dropping them, or whether or not he can, with eyes closed and arms extended, maintain his balance. These isolated facts *remain* isolated facts unless they are related to speech and language development.

For this reason, after the data pertaining to motor functions are recorded, numerous questions may be raised about the motor performance of the child, in an effort to relate this information to the child's speech and language or learning disabilities. For example, if the question is: Does the child have a problem in locomotor function, balance, dominance, or manual dexterity?, and the answer is *Yes* in any of these areas, then it must be determined to what degree the motor impairment contributes to the delayed speech and language development. If the question is: Does he have a problem in prehension, grasp, grip, or abilities to perform certain fine motor skills, boards or paper-pencil tasks?, and he *does,* then the degree to which these problems may limit his ability to participate adequately in routine classroom procedures should be explored.

There are other pertinent questions: Is there evidence of psycho-motor problems, such as tremors, tics, or bizarre, extraneous movements? If so, then some attempt should be made to determine the cause of this behavior, differentiating between possible organic or emotional etiologies. Are there any motor deviations of the lips, palate, jaws, tongue, or the articulators as a unit? If so, then the degree to which these motor problems exist, and their relationship to the child's speech and language problem, should be studied further. Is he able to vary the pitch, volume, rate, or rhythm of his voice? If not, further study of his inability to do so is indicated in order to relate his voice quality with some other problem, such as hearing loss or emotional disturbance.

After asking these and other similar questions, we may be able to assess with more accuracy answers to three basic questions about motor development: (1) How much of the child's motor behavior deviates from normal expectations? (2) What can be done to help him compensate for certain kinds of motor dysfunction; and (3) What aspects of his motor disability appear to be irreversible? In this way information about motor behavior can be related to speech and language development, and the information becomes meaning-ful to both the diagnostic and the therapeutic procedures.

AUDITORY CAPACITIES

Usually, the hearing evaluation is scheduled early in the diag-nostic sequence, because it is necessary to know whether or not a child is able to receive and comprehend auditory stimuli before his responses to other types of tests can be evaluated adequately. Hearing evaluations of the very young require special knowledge of the way in which the auditory system works and wide experience with the subtle responses of children. Because audiologic evaluations frequently are complex, the examiner may often consider the results to be merely tentative pending further observations and testing.

Because of its complexity, the audiologic examination requires the combined professional attention of the otologist and the audiologist. Some otologists and audiologists devote a major portion of their professional time exclusively to the evaluation of hearing loss in young children. One of the major responsibilities of an audiologist is to develop, adapt, and design new tests which may provide more adequate answers to the differential diagnosis of hearing loss. These techniques are tested before they are considered valid and reliable. Frequently the interpretation of results to the parents of a child with a hearing loss requires several conferences to assure their complete understanding of the problem.

81   See W. G. Hardy and others, "An Analysis of Language Development in Children with Impaired Hearing," *Acta Otolaryngologica* Supplementum 141 (1958), p. 51.

Some of the techniques used to evaluate hearing in young children are informal and cannot be described specifically. However, these procedures, when carried out by experienced and knowledgeable examiners, reveal much information about the way in which the child's auditory system functions. Some of these informal procedures may include tests requiring the imitation of vocalization, the comprehension of commands, the identification of social noises, the retention of rhythmic auditory patterns, and the response to vibration and other types of sounds found in the general environment.

82   For an interesting discussion of these informal tests, read J. O'Neill's *The Hard of Hearing* in the Prentice-Hall Foundations of Speech Pathology Series (Englewood Cliffs, N. J.: Prentice-Hall, Inc., 1964).

Other more formal tests of audition include *speech audiometry,* designed to determine at what intensity level the individual can respond to speech, both in terms of comprehension of meaning and in terms of the level at which he recognizes speech as a sound; *psychogalvanic audiometry,* based on the principle of conditioning and response and the use of *electroencephalography* to chart responses to sound, in both waking and sleeping states.

83   For information about these methods, see Carhart, Raymond, "Speech Audiometry," *Acta Otolaryngologica,* XLI (1953), No. 18; John Bordley and W. Hardy, "A Study in Objective Audiometry with the Use of a Psycho-Galvanic Response," *Annals of Otology, Rhinology, and Laryngology,* LVIII (1949), 751; and R. E. Marcus, D. L. Gibbs, and F. A. Gibbs, "Electroencephalography in the Diagnosis of Hearing Loss in the Very Young Child," *Disorders of the Nervous System,* X (1949), 170-73.

Speech and hearing specialists responsible for providing therapy for a child with delayed speech and language development or for referring children for further diagnostic work-up usually are concerned with several factors regarding the child's ability or inability to hear.

First, of course, is their concern with the evaluation of auditory acuity and the determination of the child's level of responses in terms of both intensity (db level) and frequency (cps).

84   For a detailed discussion of these and other terms pertaining to audition, see the glossary in S. S. Stevens and H. Davis, *Hearing* (New York: John Wiley & Sons, Inc., 1938), 449-56.

Second, they are concerned with whether or not the child uses the hearing he does have. Some children do not respond to sounds in their environment—at least, not at any consistent level—although no evidence can be found to support a diagnosis of hearing loss. Some of these children are unable to respond consistently to sound stimuli because of central nervous system impairment. Others apparently disregard sounds within their environment and do not respond to sound stimuli although their auditory capacities may be quite adequate.

85   See Chapter 10 in *Emotional Problems of Early Childhood,* G. Caplan, ed. (New York: Basic Books, Inc., 1955), pp. 231-47, for a case history of a child with psychogenic deafness. This unusually compelling clinical report presents a particularly interesting description of the child's temperament and expressions, p. 236.

Third, although a child may give adequate evidence of being able to hear, it is important to know whether or not he is able to *localize* the source of sound. This is particularly important in the success or failure of therapeutic procedures. The therapist can obtain some idea of the child's ability to localize sound by observing whether or not the child can locate the source of sound when a stimulus (a whistle, a bell, or a hand-clap) is presented in front of the child, behind him, and to either side. Naturally, these sounds must be presented without visual clues. This procedure, therefore, can be carried out best when the child is blindfolded or has his eyes closed or covered.

Fourth, it is important to find out whether or not the child is able to *discriminate* between two or more similar sounds. This can be done by asking him to imitate speech sounds or volume changes or rhythm changes. Social noises, which are available on recorded discs, can be used also. The procedure here is to ask the child to identify sounds either by naming them or by identifying the source of each sound by selecting the picture from several presented by the therapist, which most closely represents the source of the sound.

86   This procedure is explained in detail and the recorded discs are available in Jean Utley, *What's Its Name?, A Guide to Speech and Hearing Development* (Urbana, Ill.: University of Illinois Press, 1950).

Although these methods can be used to obtain some general idea of the child's abilities to localize or discriminate sounds, any questions about his abilities to do so should be explored through complete audiologic examination. It is not only the severe or moderate hearing losses which play havoc with a child's ability to develop speech and language; even a slight loss, when undetected, can present a major barrier to learning.

MENTAL ABILITIES

Usually, intelligence tests or scales are selected in terms of certain general qualifying factors, such as ease of administration, familiarity of the examiner with selected tests, and suitability of the testing instrument to the purpose of the examination.

Intelligence testing, with all the related intricacies of this type of examination, lies within the purview of the psychologist. Yet decisions which must be made by other specialists about a child with delayed speech and language development depend heavily upon these findings. Therefore, interpretations of these findings are, frequently, a shared responsibility. In an effort to avoid errors in the interpretation of the results of intelligence tests, it would seem pertinent to consider certain questions concerning the test procedures used to evaluate intelligence and the interpretation of findings which result from these tests. The following questions seem fairly typical:

First, why do we attempt to assess the intelligence of children with severely delayed speech and language development? Because mental subnormality is one of the major factors contributing to delayed speech and language development, it is necessary to determine a child's intellectual level when a communication problem exists. But this is not the only reason for these assessments. A primary purpose in assessing intelligence is to determine what can be done to alleviate the problem or to improve the status of children with delayed speech and language development. This implies that the examiner must weigh the child's abilities against his disabilities and his strengths against his weaknesses, and, with certain allowances for motivation, environmental factors, and similar unscorable aspects, to determine with a fair degree of confidence what each child's educational prognosis might be. Reports of intelligence testing, therefore, should provide clues for the selection of appropriate therapeutic procedures, the most effective avenues for education, and useful recommendations for parental education and guidance.

Second, why is intelligence testing of children with little or no speech such a complex and involved procedure? It is difficult enough to obtain valid test scores for children who *can* talk. We can therefore understand that evaluating the intelligence of children with limited speech and language would require even more complex procedures. Certain limitations are inherent in any attempt to evaluate the intelligence of children with little or no verbal communication. Such testing frequently depends more upon the examiner's clinical artistry than his selection and use of specific tests as isolated measurements. For example, children with severely delayed speech and language development, because of the nature of their problem, must be evaluated by using nonverbal tests. These tests consist primarily of performance-test items. The limitations imposed by the necessity for using performance tests only may not present a problem in the interpretation of tests used to evaluate very young children, because most tests used at the three-year level and below are nonverbal in nature. But tests used to evaluate older children have an increasingly higher proportion of verbal sub-tests. These exaggerate any limitation in speech and language development which might be present.

For this reason, a mentally normal child with delayed speech and language development may score at a normal level when tested at two or three years of age; but several years later, when verbal responses are required in these same test areas, he may score below normal range. Thus, if a child has received professional help with his communication problem during the interim between tests, it may appear that the major contribution of the speech and hearing therapist has been to successfully reduce the child's IQ by some 20 points. This is rather difficult to explain, particularly to parents.

Because the complexity of the test procedure is related directly to the complexity of the speech and language disorder, we tend to relegate our faith to the merits of the examiner more than to the merits of the test battery. This is as it should be. No examiner worth his certification would be content with long-term judgments based upon a single test session. At best, intelligence testing of children with communication problems can provide us only with clues. Periodic reassessments will be necessary.

Third, how useful are intelligence quotients, and what do they tell us about an individual child? IQ scores are meaningless when considered in isolation. In the evaluation of children with delayed speech and language development, the total scores are not as important as the ways in which a child attempts to solve the various test problems. Decisions about the intellectual abilities and capacities of a child with communication problems depend upon other impressions, such as the child's attitude toward the test environment; the way in which he attempts to communicate with the examiner; the degree of his success or failure on specific and divergent test items; the indications of potentially higher levels of performance; and many others. These impressions should be included in the examination report.

Fourth, what dangers are present in reporting that certain behavioral responses or physical characteristics are present? There is a tendency, at times, to attach clinical meaning to certain responses or characteristics because of a previous diagnosis or opinion. This eagerness to classify behavior can result in misleading conclusions. If a medical diagnosis of central nervous system impairment has been made, for example, this does not guarantee that the behavioral deviations sometimes associated with central problems will be present. This could result in the inaccurate classification of perseveration when it is perseverance; distractibility when it is curiosity; retardation when it is immaturity. Careless classification of physical characteristics also can lead to the erroneous classifications of problems. An example of this "jumping-to-wrong-conclusions" type of classification can be seen in the following example: Carol, a four-year-old girl, was referred by a pediatrician to the speech and hearing clinic because of a rather severe delay in speech and language development. She was a small child, with black straight hair and somewhat slanted eyes. Her pediatrician questioned, among other things, whether or not mental retardation might be the cause of her delayed speech and language development. An examiner evaluated Carol's speech and language and recommended that Carol be scheduled for a psychological examination. The examiner's report of the results from the speech and language evaluation indicated that Carol had many characteristics associated with Down's Syndrome (Mongolism), particularly her straight black hair and slanted eyes, which are physical characteristics seen frequently in Mongoloid children. The psychological report, however, indicated that Carol tested at a near-normal level and that there was no evidence to support a diagnosis of mental retardation. It later became evident that the initial examiner had been influenced unduly by the pediatrician's question concerning possible mental retardation. Through misinterpretation of the pediatric report, Carol's physical characteristics had been mis-evaluated. These facts became embarrassingly clear at the parent conference which both parents attended. Carol did not look like her blond-haired mother, but she was a female miniature of her father, who was Chinese.

This may appear to be a somewhat capricious example and one that would occur only when clinical stupidity was coupled with high suggestibility. Unfortunately, similar errors have been known to occur, some of which were not so readily tested out as this one.

Fifth, should standardized procedures be maintained in the evaluation of children with delayed speech and language development? In terms of intelligence testing, perhaps the major responsibility of the examiner who is asked to evaluate the intelligence of a child with delayed speech and language development is to make some realistic predictions concerning the child's educability. This may be where clinical artistry supersedes the use of standardized tests, given in a standardized way, with no deviation in procedure or scoring. Because standard mental tests require communication between child and examiner, a communication problem *alone* could result in the child's reduced ability to perform at maximum level. As a consequence, an erroneous diagnosis of mental retardation might be made.

87 For a discussion of which intelligence tests are most useful for children with delayed speech and language development, read W. Johnson, F. Darley, and D. C. Spriestersbach, *Diagnostic Methods in Speech Pathology* (New York: Harper & Row, Publishers, 1963), Chapter VII.

This does not mean, however, that the use of standard tests, administered in a standard way, should be avoided. Quite to the contrary! Standard procedures *must* be maintained, for one of the basic aims of any evaluation is to set down information obtained from known measurements so that the results of subsequent tests can be compared and an objective evaluation of progress obtained.

But there are two different issues here, and they must not be confused. If a standard test is used to evaluate a child with a communication problem, then the results are meaningful *only* when they are compared with the scale devised for that test. This provides us with an IQ. However, the results of standard tests should not preclude the examiner's attempt to tap all of the possible resources of a child so that a possible predictive score may also be recorded. This would provide us with a potential IQ. As long as these potential scores are interpreted as clinical impressions, these opinions may be extremely valuable in the educational planning for these children, perhaps even more valuable than a report of findings restricted to the confines of standard requirements.

In summary, we can say that, before decisions can be made about the intellectual functioning of children with delayed speech and language development, the limitations of available test instruments, the inherent complexity of the evaluation, and the dangers involved in the interpretation of test results must be recognized. Then, perhaps, we might be able to decide more selectively: *why* we are referring each child for psychologic examination; *what* we might expect the test results to indicate; and *to what extent* this information might influence our therapeutic approach to the problem.

SOCIAL MATURITY

The concept of social maturity and the measurement of social competence will not be discussed here in depth. We have chosen this plan not because a lesser value has been placed on the importance of this kind of information, but because the evaluation of social competence and the determination of social maturity are usually considered a part of the other test areas.

Maturity is not something that happens to the individual at a specific time. It cannot be dated from the day we first start to school, or can vote, or are eligible to hold office. From conception to interment, we are in the process of maturing, and what we are to become, we are in the process of becoming. Evaluation of social maturity, therefore, is concerned with ranges of development which go from dependence to independence; from incompetence to competence; from irresponsibility to responsibility.

The evaluation of social maturity is concerned with determining the individual's level of social competence. This means that we must evaluate what he does, *routinely*, to care for himself and, later, to provide care for others. We are not concerned with making judgments about what the individual *can* do on occasion, or what he *might* be able to do, if he did not have a particular problem. A child with delayed speech might be expected to have a lower social maturity quotient than a normal child simply because he cannot communicate adequately. Similarly, a child with a hearing loss will not be able to function competently in activities which will require normal hearing; a mentally retarded child will not be expected to perform adequately in tasks requiring normal intelligence; and an emotionally disturbed child will not be able to relate appropriately to activities which require a personal or social relationship with other people.

88   For a comprehensive review of social maturity and the evaluation of social competence, read *Measurement of Social Competence* (St. Louis: Educational Publishers, Inc., 1953).

EMOTIONAL STABILITY

Communication is intricately involved in the individual's need to relate to other people. Therefore, emotional stability is a major factor contributing to adequate speech and language development. Although the diagnosis of emotional problems is the responsibility of psychiatrists and psychologists, specialists from other disciplines must be able to recognize the individual who may be emotionally disturbed if they are to refer him for help with his problem. In a sense, a large number of children with delayed speech and language development may be said to have emotional problems. However, these problems in adjustment are realistic ones and occur because the child is frustrated by being unable to communicate with others. Children with central nervous system involvement, or children with hearing loss, aphasia, or other similar kinds of problems, also may have difficulty adjusting to the world around them. This may be the reason why children who have realistic or temporary difficulty adjusting because of other primary problems may be confused with children whose primary problems lie within the emotional sphere exclusively.

Speech and hearing therapists may or may not be concerned directly with children who have severe emotional disorders. However, psychiatrists and psychologists have learned to value the help of the speech and hearing therapist, for an emotionally disturbed child is even more difficult to diagnose and treat when he is limited in his ability to express himself verbally. For this reason, speech and hearing therapists may be asked to include in small stimulation groups one or two children with emotional problems. This kind of therapy has proved effective in the past, suggesting that more programs of this sort may be needed.

89 For more details about speech stimulation and the effectiveness of these procedures with emotionally disturbed children, see the excellent article by J. Tarlton Morrow, Jr., "A Psychiatrist Looks at the Non-Verbal Child," *Exceptional Children* (April 1959), pp. 347-51.

Generally speaking, children with moderate to severe emotional disorders fall within two broad categories: those considered to be neurotic and those diagnosed as psychotic. One of the points of differentiation between neurotic and psychotic symptoms is the way in which the child does or does not, can or cannot, will or will not use speech for communication purposes. This is true particularly in those children whose speech is limited to particular occasions or with particular people. The neurotic child, for example, may refuse to talk anywhere except when he is alone with his mother. Conversely, the psychotic child may make guttural sounds or vocal noises or he may yell, grunt, and use some similar vocal means of attracting attention to himself, but he usually does not use speech. If he does, it is almost certain it will not be with his mother. Emotional problems in children have been discussed in detail elsewhere, and therefore only some of the more remark-

90   Read Leo Kanner's "Irrelevant and Metaphorical Language of Early Infantile Autism," *American Journal of Psychiatry,* CIII (1946), 242-46.

able symptoms of emotional disturbance will be noted here: those limited to the more overt behavioral clues.

The two types of psychotic children who may come to the attention of the speech and hearing specialist are those with Symbiotic Psychosis or Autism, for both types have severely delayed speech and language development.

91   See Margaret Mahler's description and discussion, "On Child Psychosis and Schizophrenia," *Psychoanalytic Study of the Child* (New York: International Universities Press, 1952), VII, 286-305, for information on symbiotic psychosis. Autism is described by Leo Kanner, "Early Infantile Autism," *Journal of Pediatrics,* XXV (1944), 211-17.

Symbiotic psychosis is believed to be caused by the failure of the child to make a separation or a differentiation of his ego from that of his mother and, therefore, from the outside world. These children usually have a history of being "good" babies. As infants, they give their parents very little trouble. Usually they are quiet, placid, affectionate babies. The first symptoms of symbiotic psychosis do not begin at birth, but usually occur first when the child is two or three years of age. These symptoms frequently coincide with some occasion which threatens the separation of the child from his mother, such as illness of the child, illness of the mother, the birth of a sibling, or any other situation which separates child and mother for a fairly long period of time.

During this separation, the child may become a clinging, demanding, whining, and generally frustrated individual. However, this child must not be confused with a child who "misses" his mother because he is "attached" to her. Rather, the problems of the symbiotic child are symptomatic of a deep feeling of rejection and desertion. Hence, the child reacts as if his whole being— literally, his life—is being threatened. And, in a sense it is, because he "lives" only as long as the symbiotic relationship with his mother is maintained.

Many of these children use words, though not in the true sense of communication. Echolalia is frequent, and they may repeat phrases out of context. This repetition of phrases—even sentences— is done, apparently, without the child comprehending or understanding the meaning of them.

They also have severe difficulty with pronouns and often refer to themselves in third person at much too late a time to be considered normal—frequently as late as eight or nine years of age. They often go to great lengths to circumvent the use of the pronoun *you*, and, when they cannot avoid it any other way, they refer to "you" as *him* or *her*.

They do not play normally with toys, but instead they use them in some way which apparently makes sense to them but to no one else. Much of their behavior points to the fact that they lack the ability to form a relationship with others. They have poor eye contact. They look at people out of the corner of their eyes, or, with head bent, through the fringe of their eyelashes. They are skilled in avoiding contact with people, and can move quickly and cleverly out of range before their movements can be curtailed. They have the disconcerting knack of climbing up, running through, or jumping into extremely dangerous areas. Yet, for some reason, they seem to be able to protect themselves in these situations. They usually enjoy doing physical "tricks" and may perform unusual balance acts which might be difficult for normal children of their age. Their behavior frequently is compulsive with many routines and rituals.

Although these children cannot be accepted in the regular classroom, they seem to miss the routine of a formal education and may make unsuccessful attempts to break their own isolation. For example, they may go through the process of getting ready for school. They may gather books together and dress themselves. They may even insist on waiting for the school bus with other children. Parents of these children usually watch these procedures with total dismay and despair, one of their frequent anguished cries being: "He is ready for school. Why won't they admit him?" followed by lists of things which the child may do on occasion and which in the minds of the parents indicate that the child is capable and ready to be educated. However, it is impossible to include these children in the regular classroom—the parents know it, the teachers know it, the clinicians know it, and, perhaps, even the child knows it.

Autism

The autistic child differs from the symbiotic child in several ways; one is that he makes no relationship with anyone, not even his mother. It has been thought that perhaps his withdrawal system is partially a protective one, because he seems to have an extremely acute sensory system. Lights, sounds, smells, tastes, and tactual sensations seem to be received by his central nervous system more acutely than is expected in the normal child, and, therefore, these sensations may require a more immediate response. Although the autistic child behaves in much the same manner as the symbiotic child, the two differ in the fact that the autistic child is different almost from birth. The autistic child is *not* a "good" baby. He has sleep disturbances and formula problems, and he shows no response to the adults who care for him. He resists affection even as a young infant, either passively (he has been described as a "bag of flour") or actively (he may tense his muscles so that it is difficult to hold him in any position). He is not a "clinger"; rather, he is a "pusher away." Neurologic examinations usually reveal that he has normal neuromuscular development, and psychologic examinations may indicate that he has "unavailable" intelligence, sometimes at a superior level. The autistic child may be able to do unusual things: he may be able to hum complicated operatic arias, or he may be able to draw pictures in three dimensions. He usually uses people as he would use inanimate objects. When asked to draw a picture, he may place a pencil in the hand of the examiner and draw the picture by pushing the examiner's hand around the paper. If he leans on you, and there are occasions when he might, you represent no more to him than a wall or a lightpost. He frequently mouths objects or smells them, and he is noted for his food idiosyncrasies.

92   For further information about these unusual behavioral patterns, read
      P. Bergman and S. Excalona, "Unusual Sensitivities in Very Young
      Children," *Psycho-Analytic Study of the Child* (New York: International
      Universities Press, 1949), III, 333-52.

Most of the information related here has been discussed in more detail in the references indicated and in other descriptive writings. It is not to be assumed that any one of these behavioral clues might in isolation be indicative of severe emotional disturbance. However, the recognition of these symptoms, particularly when they occur in a cluster or a pattern, indicates the need for psychiatric and psychologic evaluation.

LANGUAGE DEVELOPMENT

Language evaluations are always done in relation to the other aspects of speech and language development: motor skills, mental abilities, auditory capacities, social maturity, and emotional stability. Viewed separately, the language evaluation can serve to summate all those components which relate to, or are responsible for, delayed speech and language development. It can be considered a prognostic tool as well as a diagnostic one. In essence, the evaluation of language development provides the speech and hearing therapist with a systematic method for recording observations of language behavior.

Examiners may differ in the procedures used to evaluate language development, but their objectives are much the same. First, the examiner must be alert to indications of the way in which the child thinks—how he perceives the world around him, how he organizes concepts, and how he formulates ideas. In terms of language development, this thinking process may be referred to as *integrative language.*

Second, the examiner is interested in how the child responds to the information he receives—whether or not he comprehends the meaning of words, and to what extent he understands what is said to him. This is referred to usually as *receptive language.*

Third, the examiner is concerned with the child's abilities to express his ideas verbally—accuracy of articulation, size of vocabulary, and complexity of sentence structure. This is called *expressive language*.

Language evaluations usually begin with an informal, nondirective, and sometimes fairly unstructured approach. The child may be brought into a room containing toys and objects of interest to children. Without too much direction, he is permitted to select those objects which are of interest to him, and the examiner records what the child does and how he behaves in this rather permissive environment. What items the child selects, and how he selects them; whether or not he plays constructively or in a meaningless manner; his use of gestures or facial grimaces to express himself; the way he arranges materials and the length of time he can occupy himself with these activities, are all of importance to the examiner.

Gradually, the examiner attempts to introduce more structure, first by manipulating objects or things in a more restrictive manner and then with an effort to have the child join him in these activities. If some type of "give and take" relationship can be established with the child, the examiner can provide more structure to play activities.

While the examiner is engaged in activities with the child, he may plan to have an observer present to record the child's responses. This eliminates any need for the examiner to rely on his memory by recording observations following the session. It is more effective if the examiner does not need to interrupt the examination and observation activities in order to record specific observations.

Toy furniture and doll figures which may represent members of the child's family or others in his environment (dolls representing the child's mother, father, sister, brother, doctor, nurse, teacher, and so forth) are used. The appropriateness of the way in which the child manipulates both furniture and dolls—the meaningfulness of the activity—gives some basis for estimating how much internal language is present and how functional this language may be for speech development. Other toys and objects also are useful: blocks, toy automobiles or airplanes, puzzles, puppets, and other similar kinds of equipment, usually familiar to the child and available to speech and hearing therapists, can be used in observing language behavior.

93   For other suggestions related to language evaluation, particularly the
      concept of "inner language," read H. R. Myklebust, *Auditory Dis-
      orders in Children* (New York: Grune & Stratton, Inc., 1954), pp. 276-89.

In the evaluation of receptive language, the procedures again
may be informal, but there is somewhat more structure to this
phase of the evaluation, because its purpose is to determine what
kinds of information the child is able to organize and comprehend
and which kinds he cannot. The child may be asked to respond
to simple commands ("Give me the doll," "Point to the ball,"
"Put the blue one here."). Then he may be asked to respond to
commands at various levels of complexity. For example, the examiner might begin with: "Come here, sit down, and draw me a
picture." If necessary, the level of complexity might be reduced
to: "Come here and sit down." If the child still cannot respond,
the command may be: "Come here," without the reinforcement of
appropriate gestures. Finally, simple commands accompanied by
gestures may be used.

Another aspect of the evaluation of receptive language has to
do with whether or not the child can judge relationships between
objects. Using objects or appropriate pictures representing them,
the examiner may ask the child to respond to questions requiring
judgments, in terms of: *size* (larger or smaller); *distance* (closer
or farther); *weight* (heavier or lighter); *volume* (empty or full);
speed (fast or slow); *length* (short or long); *time* (early or late);
and *height* (tall or short).

These and other methods devised by the examiner are used to
evaluate the way in which the child receives information and his
receptive responses to speech situations.

94   For more information about the evaluation of delayed language de-
      velopment, read Tina E. Bangs, "Evaluating Children with Language
      Delay," *Journal of Speech and Hearing Disorders*, XXVI (February
      1961), No. 1, 6-18.

The examination of *expressive* language (that is, speech) has
been discussed in some detail previously. Obviously, if the child
has speech, an articulation test can be given, and the examiner
can note which sounds are defective and in what positions (initial,
medial, or final) and to what degree they are defective, as well as
the general length of response, size of vocabulary, number of different words used, structure of sentences, and so forth.

95   For additional and detailed coverage of the evaluation of expressive language, read Chapter 7, "Appraisal of Language Development and Language Disorders," in W. Johnson, F. Darley, and D. C. Spriestersbach, *Diagnostic Methods in Speech Pathology* (New York: Harper & Row, Publishers, 1963), pp. 160-200; L. Lerea, "Assessing Language Development," *Journal of Speech and Hearing Research*, I (March 1958), 75-85; Harold Michal-Smith, and Shulamith Kastein, *The Special Child* (New School for the Special Child, Inc., Bureau of Publications, 71 Columbia Street, Seattle 4, Washington, 1963), p. 334.

Several language tests and scales are available for the evaluation of linguistic or symbolic disorders in young children which provide an opportunity for speech and hearing therapists to observe language behavior more objectively. However, there are certain factors

96   See S. Kirk, and J. McCarthy, "Illinois Test of Psycholinguistic Abilities — An Approach to Differential Diagnosis," *American Journal of Mental Deficiency*, LXVI (November 1961) No. 3; M. Crabtree, *The Houston Test for Language Development* (Houston: Houston Press, 1963), pp. 1-13.

concerning the evaluation of delayed speech and language development which remain fairly constant:

First, the evaluation of speech and language requires a multiprofessional approach. No one professional discipline is inclusive enough to provide answers to the total problem. Ideally, when a child is delayed in speech and language development, he is scheduled for a series of tests including medical, psychologic, audiologic, and speech and language evaluations. The results of all examinations are then coordinated into a single report so that final recommendations represent a cohesive approach to the problem.

Second, test items used to evaluate speech and language development may be lifted from larger test batteries, and when used in isolation or out of context, the scores must be considered inferential and highly experimental. Strides have been taken recently in the design and development of language tests and scales for children, and some of these scales provide language scores similar to intelligence quotients. In the future these tools of measurement should help to standardize examination procedures to some extent, so that results may be more comparable from clinic to clinic. However, evaluations of young children, particularly those with delayed or disturbed language development, involve a dynamic process requiring a series of test sessions over a period of time, and the interpretation of these test results must remain flexible.

Third, language evaluations, generally, are not designed to provide the examiner with absolute scores as much as they attempt to tap the child's areas of abilities as well as his disabilities, his strengths as well as his weaknesses. Hence, a major component of a speech and language evaluation is that it provides a prognostic value as well as a diagnostic one. ♫♫♫

EVALUATIONS OF DELAYED SPEECH AND LANGUAGE DEVELOPMENT DO not terminate with the completion of specific test procedures. To the contrary, it is strikingly apparent that children with delayed speech and language development frequently require long-term study in a therapeutic setting before valid diagnostic or prognostic decisions can be reached. Therefore, the speech and language therapist must be meaningfully aware of the behavioral responses which he observes daily in these children, for the study of delayed speech and language development is a dynamic and continuous process.

Certain dangers and risks are inherent in any attempt to discuss delayed speech and language development as if it were a separate entity. In fact, the entire foregoing discussion emphasizes the point

4

therapy for children with delayed speech and language development

that *delayed speech* is a broad, descriptive classification—that numerous factors can be responsible for speech and language delay. Obviously, different problems will require somewhat different therapeutic approaches. If this were not true, there would be little need to differentiate the primary problem in the first place. But before we consider some of the differences in therapeutic approach, it seems appropriate to discuss some of the more general goals, objectives, procedures, and other important aspects common to therapy for all children with delayed speech and language development.

GOALS AND OBJECTIVES

The primary goal of speech and language therapy is, of course, to help children learn to speak as accurately and as soon as possible. In addition to this primary goal, there are other objectives which may be less essential but nevertheless are important to the therapeutic process.

First is the need for therapists to be alert to clues which might indicate that a child should be referred for additional evaluation. This sometimes occurs when the results of initial tests have not been conclusive and a clear diagnostic designation cannot be assigned. In instances such as these, it frequently is the practice to schedule the child for observational therapy prior to additional examination. This period of observational therapy usually can accomplish at least two things: (1) It provides the therapist with an opportunity to observe the child's behavior over a longer period of time than is possible during diagnostic sessions. During this time the therapist can study the child's responses to a variety of stimuli and in various situations. Information resulting from observation, coupled with test evidence, may pinpoint possible problem areas. (2) Observational therapy gives the child an opportunity to become more familiar with the clinical setting before he is scheduled for additional test sessions. As he becomes better adjusted to a clinical environment, the child usually is able to respond more consistently on tasks selected by the therapist or examiner, and his abilities to perform on these tasks may begin to approximate his potential level of performance much more closely.

97   For additional discussions of the value of early education and observational or demonstration therapy, read J. Bangs, "Preschool Language Education for the Brain-Damaged Child," *The Volta Review*, LXIX (1957), 17-19; and *Speech and Language Therapy with the Brain-Damaged Child*, W. Daley, ed. (Washington, D. C.: The Catholic University of America Press, 1962).

There is another reason for referring children with delayed speech and language development for periodic evaluations, for the need for additional testing is not unique to those instances where a diagnosis has not been clearly established. Basic to the need for periodic reassessment is the inherent need to keep information about the child's progress and development current. Frequently it is difficult for a therapist who sees a child routinely to determine whether or not progress is being made in the desired areas. Although certain criteria can be developed to evaluate progress objectively, it is always helpful to obtain the opinion of another specialist, so that no possibility will be overlooked in selecting the most effective approach to the child's problem. For example, if a child has been diagnosed as mentally retarded, periodic psychologic tests will be useful; if his hearing is the primary area of question, periodic audiologic examinations will be necessary.

Usually, the shortest interval between test sessions is approximately six weeks. Naturally, the frequency of re-evaluation will depend upon the type of problem the child has and the validity of previous test results. When intelligence or another aspect of the child's mental abilities is the focal point of concern, the period between tests might range between three and six months. Physical examinations usually are scheduled at least once a year. However, specific medical examinations may be repeated at six-month intervals or even more often, depending upon what the physician advises.

Although there is no question that periodic evaluations of a child with delayed speech and language development are necessary, it is also important to realize that referring a child for additional examinations can be overdone. As a safeguard against over-referral, it is wise for the therapist to indicate why additional evaluation is considered important and what changes in the child's behavior have occurred to suggest that re-evaluation is warranted. Thus, referral planning is necessary to avoid "overtesting" the child and to prevent unnecessary expense to the parents.

A second objective of therapy and the therapeutic process is to determine more accurately the degree to which speech and language are delayed. Frequently when a child is seen over a period of time in a therapeutic setting, the nature of his problem changes in terms of both degree of involvement and prognosis. For example, during the diagnostic sequence, a child may appear to have a severe problem, and this may be an accurate appraisal of his degree of involvement at that time. However, if therapy has been effective, it is expected that the degree of involvement will have decreased, either because the problem itself has diminished, or because the child has learned to compensate for his problem to some extent. In essence, the reason for re-evaluating the child's speech and language periodically is to maintain a current picture of his progress in speech and language development and to note the changes which have occurred in his ability to communicate.

98   The importance of periodic re-evaluation of progress is noted by a
      number of writers, among them: H. Michal-Smith and S. Kastein, *The
      Special Child* (Seattle: New School for the Special Child, Inc., Bureau
      of Publications, 1963); R. L. Schiefelbusch and H. V. Bair, "Language
      Behavior of Mentally Retarded Children," *Medical Times* (September
      1960); and C. Van Riper in his chapter on delayed speech in *Speech
      Correction: Principles and Methods*, 4th Ed. (Englewood Cliffs, N. J.:
      Prentice-Hall, Inc., 1963), pp. 102-31.

A third objective of the therapeutic process is to explore the best avenues for reaching the child. Information about the child's ability to learn can be valuable to others, particularly the child's teacher and his parents. The larger goal of all therapy with young children is to help them become "ready" to be educated. The end product of speech and language therapy, therefore, is not confined to the development of speech and language. The implications of how a child responds in the therapeutic setting, whether or not he is able to learn, and of how he adapts to learning situations are all factors which are of crucial importance to his future education.

A fourth objective of speech and language therapy is to support or negate the findings of previous tests and observations. It is not unusual to find that much of the behavior described in the initial examination report may have changed considerably after the child has been in a therapeutic environment for a period of time. Part of this may be due to the child's adjustment to the clinical environment; part will be due to other maturational factors. However, the opposite has been known to occur also. Thus, a child who has been described as being extremely cooperative in a test situation may be completely uncooperative in a' therapeutic one. Because of these inconsistencies, all changes in status should be recorded, so that the history of the child may remain current, and so that the implications of the changes in behavior can be assessed.

A fifth objective of therapy may be to determine the child's prognosis for adequate speech and language development. Frequently in a test situation, a child may appear to have a *poor* or a *guarded* prognosis for speech and language development, as determined by his performance on various tests in the diagnostic battery. Yet, he may be found to perform in a therapeutic setting at a much higher level than these test results suggest. Conversely, some children may be expected to have fairly good potential, yet they do not make the predicted gains in speech and language acquisition. When this occurs, of course, it is necessary to determine whether the lack of progress is due to an ineffective therapeutic approach or to an inaccurate prognostic estimate. In any event, the prognosis is a necessary component of the therapeutic planning for children with delayed speech and language development. In fact a diagnosis without a careful consideration of prognostic implications has negligible value.

99   Predictive values are discussed in C. W. Pettit, "The Predictive Efficiency of a Battery of Articulatory Diagnostic Tests," *Speech Monographs,* XXIV (1957), 219-26.

In addition to the foregoing objectives, one of the most important goals of therapy is to gather additional information about the child, not only from observation of his behavior and responses in a therapeutic setting, but also from periodic conferences with the child's parents, as therapy progresses. It is not unusual for parents to omit important information during the initial diagnostic sessions, either because they are unaware of the possible significance of the information or because they are so concerned about their child's welfare at the time that they momentarily "forget" important informational items. However, as the child's therapy sessions become an expected part of the family schedule, and as the parents become more relaxed because "something is being done" about their child's problem, additional information is frequently forthcoming. For example, parents may have "forgotten" to report that their child is receiving drugs or other medication. Or, although medication has been prescribed for the child, the parents may have decided not to follow the physician's recommendation. All of this unreported information can have a direct bearing on the way in which the therapist approaches the child's problem.

Parents also have been known to "forget" to report that their child is receiving help from other sources at the same time that he is scheduled for speech and language therapy. In some instances, the child may be receiving psychotherapy, occupational therapy, or physical therapy, or he may be being tutored at the same time that he is being seen by a speech and language therapist. This combined approach to a problem, in itself, presents no problem. In fact, a composite approach is encouraged, so long as each specialist involved knows what other services the child is receiving. Without this knowledge, one therapist may unknowingly be canceling out the effectiveness of another. Only through cooperative and cohesive planning can a child benefit from various types of help simultaneously.

In addition, it is also possible that other members of the child's family, perhaps the parents themselves, might be receiving treatment of some sort, and the results of such treatment may have some direct effect on the child who is receiving speech and language therapy. This brings to mind the story about the distraught mother who visited the psychiatrist because her little boy was so difficult to manage at home. She was so upset and disturbed that the psychiatrist, instead of examining her child at that time, gave the mother a prescription for tranquilizers and told her to take two a day for three weeks and to return to the office at that time to have her child examined. Three weeks later the mother returned to the psychiatrist's office alone. "Well, Mrs. Blodgit," said the psychiatrist, "where is Billy, and how has he been getting along?" Mrs. Blodgit smiled in a relaxed and vague manner and responded, "Who cares?"

One final objective of therapy might be mentioned here: the therapeutic setting is used also to determine individual levels of achievement for each child with delayed speech and language development. Actually, it is through the therapeutic procedures, probably more than through the diagnostic process, that realistic clinical goals for each child can be established. Only by establishing realistic goals can the child's progress be evaluated objectively, so that therapy sessions will not be continued past productivity. One of the major problems which occurs all too frequently is that therapy is a shotgunned process, with little or no concern for near-term or long-term goals. This less-than-satisfactory approach occurs when the therapist is unprepared, and an unprepared therapist does little more than baby-sit. Undoubtedly, the best-conceived therapy plans cannot be followed at times, particularly if the child is very young. However, both near-term and long-term goals and aims must be set down clearly and realistically if the approach to a problem is to be effective.

In summary, the primary objectives of therapy for children with delayed speech and language development include the following: to help children develop adequate speech as soon as possible; to refer children for further examination when the need is indicated; to determine the degree of involvement present in each child; to explore the avenues considered best for reaching each child; to support or negate specific test findings and observations; to determine prognosis; to obtain information about the child for counseling and guiding his parents; and to determine realistic goals and aims for each child.

FACILITIES, EQUIPMENT, AND MATERIALS

In the not too distant past, speech and hearing therapists could be found working in most any type of facility. On occasion therapy has been scheduled in boiler rooms of schools, in linen rooms of hospitals, and under stairwells of clinics. Perhaps some very effective speech and language therapy has been carried out in facilities of this sort. However, there is little question that a therapy room which is conducive to learning — one that is bright, cheerful, but not cluttered — adds measurably to the therapeutic process.

The size of the room is of importance, particularly when working with small children. It is advantageous to have a room that is large enough to hold a group of six or eight children, but not so large that the children become disorganized when they are in it. The area should be relatively free from excess noise and should have furniture that is appropriate in size and function for young children. An observation room with a two-way-vision mirror, adjoining the therapy room, is very useful. While seated in the observation room, parents and other specialists involved with the welfare of the child can observe him without interrupting the therapy session. The observation room should, of course, be wired for sound reception, so that the observer can hear, as well as see, the child.

Equipment used for speech and language therapy does not necessarily require a large investment of money, nor is an expensive amount of equipment required. Certainly, the therapist should have access to an audiometer and a tape recorder, and it may be advantageous also to have a disc recorder available so that permanent records of samples of the child's speech at various times can be recorded. Certain test equipment, such as form boards used in perceptual training, a telebinocular used to test binocular vision, a tachistoscope which can be used for evaluating speed and accuracy in visual perception, and other similar types of equipment can be extremely useful. However, these equipment items are not mandatory for good therapy.

By the same token, therapy materials are required in both abundance and variation. Recently a speech therapist was asked to take inventory of the materials she usually carried from therapy session to therapy session. She placed on a table the following items: a fishing game, a pack of cards with rabbits and ducks and other animals on them, a box of crayons, a stack of paper, some big pencils, several *Life* magazines, articulation test blanks, and a flannel board. In addition, she had several puzzles, blocks, balls, jacks, gold stars for rewards, art paper, and gum erasers. For some time she had saved the cardboard backs of tablets, on which she had pasted selected pictures from the *Ladies' Home Journal* and similar magazines. Under each of these pictures she had printed the appropriate names: *boat, boy, dog,* and so forth. For language therapy, she had a collection of toy animals, doll figures, toy automobiles, toy airplanes, whistles, bells, colored yarn, and clay. And, as one will find almost without fail in a speech therapist's materials, she had a legal-size pad of yellow paper for taking notes and for keeping therapy logs. Having recently read some of the literature on dysarthria and cerebral palsy, she had some peanut butter and some cereal, which could be placed on various parts of a child's mouth as a stimulus for motor-kinesthetic training of tongue movements.

100   For more information regarding speech therapy for children with severe motor dysfunction of the articulators, see H. Westlake, *A System for Developing Speech with Cerebral Palsied Children* (Chicago: National Society for Crippled Children and Adults, 1951).

She also had some chalk, finger paints, paste, and art paper. Because this therapist worked in a public school system, she carried a map showing the various schools for which she provided speech and hearing therapy and the days in the week she was expected at each school.

A young man who was a staff member at a university clinic also was asked about the materials he used in therapy. His list of materials was much the same — a few more tongue blades, perhaps, but otherwise very similar. It was found that therapists who work in a hospital setting usually have more materials for work with adults than for work with children, but the items are similar in type if not in quantity. In general, it seems that clinics or hospital settings make fewer demands on speech therapists in terms of carrying materials from place to place, but no less demand on the need to create interesting ways to stimulate responses from individuals with communication disorders. Thus, anyone who has observed the amount and kinds of materials which a speech and hearing therapist gathers together over a period of a few years would be convinced that, in addition to being in excellent physical condition in order to transport these various materials, a speech therapist must be imaginative, creative, and vitally interested in the job which must be done.

We may jest somewhat about the amounts and types of materials frequently found in a speech therapist's panoply, but it should be very clear that the materials themselves are not the focal point of this discussion. Rather, it is the clinical knowledge of the therapist — his imagination, creativity, and therapy skill — which makes these materials useful.

There are, however, a few points about the materials themselves which should be noted:

First, materials should be kept in some systematic order — Fibber McGee's closet has no place in a clinical setting. Materials might be organized in terms of developmental levels, chronological ages, or areas of use, such as those used for visual, auditory, and tactual stimulation. They should be cross-indexed in some way so that the intended use is indicated but not required. A systematic storing plan eliminates last-minute searching for materials to be used and provides an ongoing inventory of available materials which makes plans for future purchases much more efficient.

Second, materials used in therapy should be kept in good repair, with no parts missing or broken. When we use materials which are incomplete or not in good working order, we increase the child's basic confusion and reduce his motivation and response. Hence, inadequate or inappropriate materials do nothing to increase the effectiveness of therapy.

Third, materials used in therapy should be well-constructed and able to resist the wear and tear of young children. Anything that is easily breakable can be potentially dangerous to a young child. Sharp edges, springs, metal rims, small, removable parts, and paint which is toxic should be avoided.

101 An excellent discussion of the use of materials designed for use in the Montessori Method of teaching can be found in Sylvia O. Richardson, *Early Teaching for Children with Minor Central Nervous System Dysfunction* (New York: United Cerebral Palsy Association, 1964).

Briefly, the facilities needed for speech and language therapy should be conducive to learning and appropriate in size for young children. Although the therapeutic process does not demand the extensive amount of equipment required for diagnostic procedures, access to an audiometer and a tape recorder is necessary. Materials should be carefully selected, stored in some systematic order, and conscientiously kept in good repair.

THERAPEUTIC PROCEDURES AND APPROACH

As would be expected, the procedures used in speech and language therapy vary from therapist to therapist and from child to child. There are, nevertheless, some broad philosophical points which apply to the selection of procedures and techniques while the approach to the child's speech and language problem is being planned.

At the outset of therapy, time must be spent on evaluating each child in various areas of development so that a clear picture of his abilities as well as of his disabilities can be established. It is a basic educational premise that children do not learn through their disabilities or weaknesses, but rather through a reinforcement of their abilities and strengths. Therefore, in our approach to children with

102 The educational needs of children with various problems are discussed at length in W. Cruickshank and G. O. Johnson, *Education of Exceptional Children and Youth* (Englewood Cliffs, N. J.: Prentice-Hall, Inc., 1958). Also read N. E. Wood, "Educational Evaluation of School Aged Children with Language Disorders," in *Speech and Language Therapy with the Brain-Injured Child*, W. Daley, ed. (Washington, D. C.: Catholic University of America Press, 1963).

delayed speech and language development, we must ascertain what the child *can* do and, through these strengths and abilities, approach the areas in which he has difficulty.

It is equally important to develop some objective criteria for evaluating the child's progress during therapy, so that therapy sessions are not continued past his current ability to benefit from them. No child will learn at a continuous rate or at a constant

level. Because time is required to absorb new information, occa-
sional clinical vacations may be necessary. By establishing unbiased
criteria for the evaluation of progress, the therapist can determine
when these clinical vacations are needed and what changes in development might be expected to transpire during the suggested
vacation from therapy. The details of the recommendation should
be explained to the parents so that they may understand clearly the
role they must assume as they observe their child during this interim.

Generally speaking, the therapeutic approach to children with
delayed speech and language development should be carried out
quietly, surely, and warmly, but without an overpowering attack.
Some therapists act as if therapy is something that is done *to* a
child, but the therapist who engulfs a child only manages to confuse
him. Progress is a growing thing; it takes time for the therapist to
become acquainted with the child. Even more important, it takes
time for the child to respond to new situations, as well as to an
adult who is totally strange to him. A child should have an opportunity to demonstrate what he can do, what he likes to do, and what
he has been successful in doing. His interests and success can be
used as a wedge to lead him through those activities and skills
which the therapist wants him to master.

Speech and language therapy should start with activities which
approximate the level at which the child is operating at the time,
or even somewhat below it. Because the child will not be able to
perform in all types of functions with equal competence, the therapist should begin with some activities which the child can do with
ease, coupled with some that he is just beginning to master.

In order to accomplish this, materials should be selected which
are appropriate to the age of the child. It is important, also, to use
equipment and techniques pertinent to the individual child's problem rather than those which merely happen to be available or to use
certain techniques only because they have been successful with
other children having similar problems.

> 103   Compare the materials and techniques suggested in the two books:
> M. McGinnis, *Aphasic Children* (Washington, D. C.: The Volta Bureau,
> 1963), and H. Barry, *The Young Aphasic Child* (Washington, D. C.:
> The Volta Bureau, 1961).

Therapy becomes more cohesive if the therapist plans some activities which can be continued at home by the child's parents, with

full realization that the child's mother cannot act in the capacity of therapist or teacher for her own child, regardless of how objective she might be. Because the child will probably be in the clinic or center a very small portion of the day, and usually only once a week, it is necessary to guide the parents so that therapy can be reinforced and substantiated at home. Toward this goal, it may be possible for the parents to duplicate some of the equipment and materials used in therapy sessions.

In brief, therapy should be planned in such a way that the child begins to anticipate these sessions with interest, pleasure, and a desire to learn. If the child learns to look forward to therapy, separation problems will be at a minimum. Parents should be urged to prepare for their child's therapy session. Children who are rushed through traffic to meet an appointment or dragged into the therapy room wailing and screaming are not in any condition to learn. It is extremely important that these children have a routine established for them both at home and in therapy which is planned and organized in such a way that a learning climate is created to which the child can attach meaning.

RECORDS AND PROGRESS REPORTS

One of the most time-consuming responsibilities of the speech and language therapist, and, perhaps, one of the most important aspects of therapy, is record-keeping and the maintenance of progress reports. The therapist who, week after week, reports vague information, such as: "Worked on *b* and *p* today. Will work on *b* and *p* again next time," falls far short of what is necessary for good therapy records, because such notations have only vague meaning for the therapists who may have the child assigned to them subsequently, or for the examiners who may be scheduled to examine the child at a later date.

One way to approach the preparation of more comprehensive records and reports would be to pose certain questions and, then, answer these questions in the report of progress. A few examples of the kinds of questions which might lend themselves to record-keeping are: Can the child make a selected sound or sounds in isolation? Can he imitate the therapist's production of these sounds?

Can he recall how the sounds should be made from therapy session to therapy session? Can he join new sounds with the sounds he is beginning to master? What is the best avenue for approaching him — through the visual, tactual, or auditory senses? In what therapy tasks is he successful? What materials does he find most interesting? Is the mother able to work with him effectively at home? Does he seem to benefit from the reinforcement of work at home? What appears to be the best over-all approach to his delayed speech and language development? Why was this approach selected instead of others? Answers to these and other similar questions give some basis for progress evaluations. Charts and graphs of progress can be helpful also. In any event, some method of assigning objective

104   One such chart is described in Ruth Anderson's article, "Report on the Development of a Communicative Evaluation Chart," ASHA, VI (1964), 81-83.

values to the child's progress is a necessary and valuable part of the total therapeutic process.

In general, then, progress reports should contain some statement of goals and intentions of therapy. Records of progress and methods for re-evaluation are necessary parts of the total therapeutic process. Progress reports should give a clear indication of both near- and long-term goals, and a careful report of the procedures used to obtain these objectives should be included in the case history.

PARENT CONFERENCES

Parents, by their own admission, are a strange breed. Talk with them about their own health problems, the rising cost of living, even the far-reaching implications of nuclear warfare, and the typical parent can discuss these subjects objectively and with detached emotion. But talk with them about a problem which their child has, and, more frequently than not, they become not only less objective but at times irrational.

When a child has a problem, parents frequently try to place the blame somewhere. They may blame the doctors, they may blame the hospitals, they may blame the schools. Most often, however, they blame themselves. Even after the child has been examined thoroughly and his problem has been discussed fully with his parents; even when the child is receiving help with his problem, his parents may still be confused and tormented, asking over and over again, "Why did this have to happen to us?"

Because of this confusion and unleashed wrath, parents are unable at times to make wise judgments about their child. They argue at home about what should be done to help their child, vacillating from one opinion to another. One day they are strict disciplinarians; the next day they are maudlin and permissive. At one time they follow professional advice to the letter; then they may follow this by a total disregard for all recommendations.

The most formidable enemy of all parents is the feeling of guilt. When a child has a problem which requires a series of examinations, parents may feel guilty for "subjecting" their child to various test situations. However, they also feel guilty if they do not make every effort to have the testing completed. Parents usually feel guilty if, after having their child examined at one clinic, they take the child to another clinic for evaluations. Yet they feel guilty, also, if they do not take advantage of every possible solution to their child's problem. They feel guilty if they pay undue attention to their child with a problem, especially if it appears that they are not equally attentive to his siblings. But they feel guilty also if they do not, in some way, show this child that they love him in spite of his problem.

Parents react to their child's problem with guilt, frustration, and confusion for one simple reason — they are human beings. All of us respond to problems we cannot solve in much the same manner, but the reactions of parents are intensified by the feeling of total inadequacy to help another human being for whom they alone are responsible.

Because these responses are a natural part of parenthood and, therefore, are to be expected, and because, in the final analysis, the parents alone are responsible for their child's welfare, parent conferences unquestionably are a vital part of the therapeutic and educational process. Any speech and language therapist who at-

105   For information along these dimensions, with particular concern for the brain-injured child, read R. Barsch, "Counseling the parent of the brain damaged child," *Journal of Rehabilitation* (May-June 1961), **27**, 26-27, 40-42, and R. Lewis, A. A. Strauss, and L. E. Lehtinen, *The Other Child:*

The *Brain-Injured Child* (New York: Grune & Stratton, Inc., 1960). Suggestions for parents of children with various speech and language disorders can be found in an interesting discussion written by C. Van Riper in *Your Child's Speech Problems* (New York: Harper and Row, Publishers, 1961).

tempts to work with a child without periodic conferences with the child's parents must be satisfied to work in a vacuum.

There are times, however, when a sound clinical relationship between therapist and parents has not been or cannot be established. In situations such as these, it is necessary to analyze critically why a less than satisfactory parent-therapist relationship exists.

One reason given for the infrequent scheduling of parent conferences is that they require too much time. This is a poor excuse. A much longer period of time may be necessary if a child is scheduled for therapy without the parents' understanding and support. Therapists in public school systems sometimes report that school regulations do not permit the scheduling of parent conferences with school personnel other than school administrators or classroom

106   Read, Martha Black, *Speech Correction in the Schools* in the Prentice-Hall Foundations of Speech Pathology Series (Englewood Cliffs, N. J.: Prentice-Hall, Inc., 1964).

teachers. Yet speech therapy cannot be an activity that is considered ancillary to the child's education. Any child who has a speech and language problem severe enough to warrant professional attention also has a problem severe enough to require interpretation and professional discussions of his problem with his parents. There are those occasions, of course, where the therapist finds that it is not possible to communicate with or "reach" a particular set of parents. This is not a unique situation, for one of the first rules that a speech therapist must learn is that no one can be all things to all people, and that no individual will be able to respond positively to all children or to all parents. Yet, some method must be devised to take care of these situations when they arise. Obviously, the most immediate solution is to schedule the child with another therapist, but this is not always possible or really necessary. Sometimes a breakthrough in communication occurs, both with unreachable parents and with intolerable children, when they are scheduled for conferences or therapy in a group. Group therapy and group parent conferences have been known to provide at least a partial answer to some of these problems.

But even when a strong clinical relationship between a therapist and a child's parents has been established, a breakdown in the communication system may occur. This break in a previously satisfactory relationship might be caused by a number of factors:

First, parents sometimes have a tendency to become too dependent, particularly when their dependency is encouraged. They may ask the therapist to help them solve problems or make decisions, many of which have nothing to do with their child's speech and hearing problem. Some therapists, either because they believe they are "needed" or because they misevaluate their own competence, may attempt to play oracle by actively participating in all of the family's problem-solving, question-answering pursuits. Usually, the therapist fails in this all-inclusive role, and the parents may begin to question his competence even in the areas where his advice is professionally sound. The wise therapist, therefore, avoids being placed in such a position of prophet or soothsayer, and he makes every effort to help parents maintain a role which is cooperatively independent. To do this, the therapist knows that a warm, interested relationship with both parents and child is more effective when coupled with a certain clinical aloofness.

Second, parents may be permitted to observe therapy prematurely, without being told what to expect or without understanding the aims and goals of the therapeutic process. Observation of therapy without explanation can lead to at least two problems: (1) Parents may attempt to imitate at home what they have observed in therapy, without understanding the procedures or without knowing what to expect from the child; or (2) Because subconsciously they have expected miracles, parents may become disenchanted with the day-by-day labor of therapy and lose confidence in the therapist when these expected miracles do not take place.

To reduce the possibility of either of these misunderstandings occurring, the therapist should discuss the child's problem with the parents both in terms of what needs to be done and in terms of how the therapist intends to approach the child's problem.

Third, parent-therapist communication can become limited if the parents feel intimidated by the therapist. For example, suppose that the parents would like to take their child to another clinic for examination, but they hesitate to discuss this idea because they are afraid of the therapist's response or because they want to avoid another lecture on "clinical shopping." As a result of this intimidation, either they will maintain an undercurrent of resentment toward the therapist, or they will take the child to the other clinic without the therapist's knowledge. Either way, the child loses. The therapist, therefore, must make it clear to parents, through actions as well as words, that their ideas about their child are always welcomed, and that, in the final analysis, the parents alone are responsible for the welfare of their child.

Finally, communication between therapist and parents may become measurably reduced as therapy progresses. This may occur because the therapist routinely uses the entire conference time to "inform" the parents of how their child is progressing in therapy, and to "discuss" what additional objectives need to be reached. However, parent conferences are a "two-way street," and on occasion it may be a more valuable and meaningful use of time to have the parents do most of the "informing" and "discussing." This may be the only opportunity the parents have to discuss their child's problem from their vantage point. Therefore, the therapist must be a good listener as well as a good informant.

In summary, parent conferences assume a major role in all therapeutic and educational processes. A therapist who attempts to provide help for a child without periodic conferences with the child's parents imposes an unnecessary limitation to the child's progress. There is a need for a sound clinical relationship between the therapist and the child's parents if parents are to be instrumental in making the therapeutic process more effective.

107   For an interesting discussion of parent discussions and parent conferences, read E. McDonald, *Understand Those Feelings* (Pittsburgh: Stanwix House, Inc., 1962).

DIFFERENCES IN THERAPEUTIC APPROACH

The foregoing discussion has been concerned with some of the more general goals, objectives, procedures, and other aspects of therapy which are common to the work with all children with delayed speech and language development. But, because several major clinical problems are presented by children with delayed speech and language development, each problem requires a somewhat different therapeutic emphasis. The discussion which follows describes some of the common varieties of problems which frequently confront the speech and hearing therapist in schools, clinics, and hospitals. No attempt will be made to discuss specific techniques or approaches to these problems. However, pertinent references throughout the discussion should provide adequate suggestions for further exploration at the reader's convenience. It should be noted, also, that the descriptions which follow are presented with the full realization that no child is representative of all children who fall within a particular diagnostic category, and that the behavior described cannot be expected to occur in all children with the same or a similar problem.

CENTRAL NERVOUS SYSTEM IMPAIRMENT

Although the term *central system impairment* may be academically correct, it does little to describe the type of child we are concerned with here. Yet other terms—"brain-injured child," "minimal brain damage," "neurophrenia," "psychoneurological learning disabilities," "Strauss syndrome" — have not met with universal acceptance. What all of these terms attempt to describe is the child

108 For a further discussion of these terms and other problems connected with terminology, read C. R. Strothers' interesting discussion, *The Neurologically Handicapped Child* (Chicago: National Society for Crippled Children and Adults, 1963).

who, because of damage to the brain, demonstrates all or some of certain behavioral characteristics which differentiate his problem from other problems resulting from cerebral damage, such as cerebral palsy and mental retardation. His lack of speech development or, more accurately, his inability to communicate ideas is, of course, just one part of his total problem.

From an educational standpoint, one of the major problems which these children have lies in the sphere of emotional behavior. Because of their inability to conform behaviorally to school requirements, they usually are excluded from the regular classroom. More generally speaking, a child with central nervous system impairment may have difficulties in several spheres: he may have a motor problem; he may have a disturbance in percept and concept formation;

he may have a severe language disability, including an inability to comprehend or use symbols for communication which are necessary for speech, reading, or writing; he may be hyperactive and distractible, lacking the ability to conform behaviorally to generally accepted social and emotional standards.

> 109 For additional information concerning these areas of disturbance, read R. S. Lewis's *The Other Child: The Brain-Injured Child*, Rev. Ed. (New York: Grune & Stratton, Inc., 1960).

In the extreme, the "brain-injured" child is not difficult to identify behaviorally, for he stands out in any clinical setting as being remarkably different. The account which follows describes some of the responses of one child who is fairly representative of this particular diagnostic category.

> 110 For additional information concerning these children, read A. A. Strauss and L. E. Lehtinen, *Psychopathology and Education of the Brain-Injured Child* (New York: Grune & Stratton, Inc., 1947).

Paul was physically well developed and difficult to restrain. He seldom entered a room — he invaded it. He walked as if his shoes were two sizes too large for him, and he loped and lunged down hallways, not unlike a Saint Bernard out for a long-belated airing. Paul seemed to notice everything. Yet he looked at objects without really seeing them. He would look intently at bulletin boards, drinking fountains, wastebaskets, lights, elevators — almost everything and anything within his environment. His looking was accompanied usually by constant, frantic motions, as if he were searching for something which might in some way, have specific meaning for him. Although his explorations were done methodically, they were carried out without any obvious reaction on his part, like an absent-minded ritual.

His motor organization was different, too. He could climb a jungle gym in his clumsy, overreaching style and stand poised on the top rung while the adults around him frantically begged him to come down. This combination of clumsiness and intricate balance was typical of his motor behavior. And yet, after performing feats of balance such as these, he might climb down from his perch and fall over a piece of chalk or crayon on the floor. His hyperactivity and constant movement were one of the major concerns of his parents. It was obvious that this constant movement would have to be curtailed in some way if Paul was to benefit from any learning situation.

> 111 A control of hyperactivity has been studied in considerable depth during the last ten years, and the need for *structure* in a therapeutic setting has been emphasized. For more information about a structured approach to brain-injured children, read W. Cruickshank and others, *A Teaching Method for Brain-Injured and Hyperactive Children*, Special Education and Rehabilitation Monograph, Series 6, Syracuse University Press, Box 87, University Station, Syracuse 10, New York. This monograph contains reports on research concerning the effect of certain teaching methods and environmental changes on brain-injured and hyperactive children. It emphasizes programming in the areas of training. Also see O. E. Hood, *Your Child or Mine; the Brain-Injured Child and His Hope* (New York: Harper & Row, Publishers, 1957), p. 180, for a discussion of the brain-injured child in a private, residential school. For additional references about work with these children, write to the National Society for Crippled Children and Adults, Chicago, Illinois, for the selected annotated references concerned with brain injury and related disorders in children.

In additon to his hyperactivity, Paul was highly distractible. Usually, the slightest sound — the turning of pages in a book, typing sounds, the dropping of a small object on the floor, even the sound from fluorescent lighting — would cause him to stop what he was doing and attempt to find the place where the sound originated. Movements also distracted him — if someone moved to pick up an object, or if a door opened suddenly, or if the wind moved the trees — these and similar slight movements seemingly compelled him to stop what he was doing and attempt to find the source of the movement.

Incongruously, with all this attention to inconsequential stimuli, Paul was able to tolerate sounds at an intensity level far above what was normally expected. He had been observed to sit in a soundproof room where pure tones were presented at more than a 90-decibel level, without so much as a blink of an eye or a turn of his head.

Other indications of perceptual difficulties could be seen also. For example, although Paul was able to identify a straight-line drawing when the picture was presented against a plain background, he was unable to identify the same picture when it was presented against a background which had a design.

112   This difficulty in differentiating a figure from a background has been studied in considerable detail. For a more complete discussion of figure-ground disturbances, and other perceptual disorders, read A. A. Strauss and N. C. Kephart, *Psychopathology and Education of the Brain-Injured Child, II: Progress in Theory and Clinic* (New York and London: Grune & Stratton, Inc.). For methods used to evaluate visual perception, refer to G. N. Getman and N. C. Kephart, *Advanced Tests of Visual Perception* (Loveland, Colorado: Childcare Co., 1953).

Paul had developed speech, but he failed to communicate ideas through speech. He usually talked at inappropriate times and on inappropriate subjects. He might begin with a specific idea, which he apparently wished to discuss, but his speech would wander away from the subject and he would include things which had occurred in the past, or objects which he had seen in his surroundings, or people's names which he seemed to remember suddenly. His conversation sounded something like this: "I saw a dog — ah — the chalk mama put to the desk — ah — on the picture pinned there — have you seen the car? My name is Paul; I am eight years old. Goodbye."

In essence, Paul's problem, like those of other children classified in this category, can be described generally under three major headings: disturbances in concept formation and perception, disturbances in motor coordination and behavior, and disturbances in language.

113   More details about these three problem areas can be found in Lauretta Bender, *Psychopathology of Children with Organic Brain Disorders* (Springfield, Ill.: Charles C. Thomas, Publisher, 1956).

The most common characteristics of children like Paul are hyperactivity, distractibility, perseveration, motor incoordination, disturbances of percept and concept formation, and disorders of language, all of which occur in varying degrees. Hence, the varieties of children classified as "brain-injured" on the basis of these characteristics could range from the child who is uncontrollable, unreachable, unpredictable, and totally unmanageable to the child whose language problem centers around his inability to use tenses of verbs correctly. Because many of these children are referred for speech and language therapy, regardless of degree of involvement, speech and language therapists must arrive at some basic philosophy about these children, their problems, and the role which they, as therapists, can assume in the total approach to the habilitation of these children. Following are a few points which might be considered in this process.

First, these children require a total educational approach, and speech and language therapy is only one part of their total needs. The speech and language therapist who takes on the total responsibility for the habilitation and education of a child with central nervous system impairment is assuming more responsibility than any one specialist should.

> 114   For additional comments along this dimension, read C. R. Strother, *Neurologically Handicapped Child* (Chicago: National Society for Crippled Children and Adults, Inc., 1963).

Second, when hyperactivity and distractibility are present to the degree that the child is unable to attend to the task at hand, it is necessary to control this behavior to a great extent before the child can benefit from a learning situation. This may necessitate considerable structure in the therapeutic setting. This means that therapy should be scheduled in a room with carpeted floors, sound-treated walls and ceilings, and without windows, pictures on the walls, or toys or equipment which are not in use.

Also, the advisability of a fairly rigid routine has been fairly well tested out, and it has been suggested that, from the time the child enters the classroom or therapy room until the time he leaves it, he should know generally what is expected of him in terms of routine.

> 115   Further discussion of the need for routine can be found in N. C. Kephart's *The Brain-Injured Child in the Classroom* (Chicago: National Society for Crippled Children and Adults, 1963).

However, the therapist must also realize that it is necessary to prepare this child to live in a world which is far from structured. Both of these concepts — structure in the therapeutic setting and total lack of structure outside the therapeutic setting — are contrasting elements which should concern the therapist as therapy progresses.

Third, the speech and language therapist must also deal with the concept of early detection of problems and early therapy as a prevention of secondary disabilities. There is reason to believe that, if these children can be scheduled for therapy at an early age, some secondary problems such as frustrations, hyperactivity, and distractibility might be diminished, if not avoided. Although working

116   This point is developed further in A. A. Strauss, "The Education of the
       Brain-Injured Child," *American Journal of Mental Deficiency,* LVI
       (1951), 712-18.

with these children as early as possible is an important point to
consider, the therapist must realize also that these children will not
benefit measurably from therapy scheduled one-half hour once a
week. Because they depend on routine to anchor them in a world
which is spinning too fast for them, therapy for these children
should be on a daily basis.

Fourth, the speech and language therapist who works with brain-
damaged children needs special professional preparation in addition
to developing a unique tolerance for the behavior of these children.
The teacher or therapist who works with these children must have
a thorough knowledge of child development, as well as special preparation in speech and language development and an understanding
of the basic educational concepts, such as those involved in teaching
reading, writing, and arithmetic. In addition, the therapist who
works with these children must be thoroughly grounded in the differential diagnosis of speech and language disorders in children.
Awareness of behavior patterns and the meaning of these responses,
as well as a knowledge of the psychiatric implications of the behavior of these children, is of utmost importance.

117   For additional information concerning this point, read L. Eisenberg,
       "Psychiatric Implications of Brain Damage in Children," *Psychiatric
       Quarterly,* XXXI (1957), 72.

APHASIA

Although children with aphasia may also have disturbances in
concept formation and perception, as well as disturbances in motor
coordination and behavior, the focal point of their educational
problem lies within the area of language disability. Aphasia in

118   For additional information about language disorders and clues for
       the identification of these problems, read K. de Hirsch, "Gestalt
       Psychology as Applied to Language Disturbances," *Journal of Nervous
       and Mental Disease,* CXX (1954), 257-61; and O. Solnitzky, "Disturb-
       ances of Language Formulation and Expression," *General Practice,*
       XIV (1956), 83-94. A contrast is drawn between problems of aphasia
       and alexia in the article written by N. E. Wood, "Language Disorders:
       Major Barriers to Communication," *School Life,* XLIII (June 1961).

children has received considerable attention during the last decade, but it is not a new problem by any means. Since the problems of

119   Read A. W. G. Ewing, *Aphasia in Children* (London: Oxford University Press, 1930). For more recent articles on the same subject, read H. R. Myklebust, "Aphasia in Children: Language Development and Language Pathology," in L. Travis, *Handbook of Speech Pathology* (New York: Appleton-Century-Crofts, Inc., 1957); A. A. Strauss, and E. N. McCarus, "A Linguist Looks at Aphasia in Children," *Journal of Speech and Hearing Disorders*, XXIII (1958), 54-58; and N. E. Wood, "The Child with Aphasia," *The Journal Lancet*, LXXIX (July 1959), 315-17.

aphasia may vary considerably from child to child, both in degree of involvement and in type of language disability, perhaps a description of one child classified as having aphasia would be helpful here.

If one word were selected to describe children with aphasia, that word would be *confused*. Dennis was a good example of this particular kind of confusion. He was unable to follow simple commands or directions, unable to match colors, unable to assemble puzzles or form boards adequately, unable to sort objects into common groups, and generally unable to perform adequately on any task which required organization. Like Paul, Dennis was distractible on many occasions, particularly when unpredicted movement or light changes occurred. On rare occasions he seemed to respond to sounds in his environment, but these responses were inconsistent and infrequent. Either his facial expression was one of questioning, with furrowed brows and an intense look, or, completely to the contrary, his expression might be totally blank, as if a veil had dropped between him and all that surrounded him. He had periodic temper tantrums, frequently unrelated to any of the activities which were going on about him at the time. His temper tantrums

120   For additional information concerning the difficulties children with aphasia have in adjusting to their surroundings, read R. Meyers and M. Meyers, "Adjustment Problems of the Aphasic Child," *The Crippled Child*, XXVIII (April 1951).

and emotional outbursts seem to be related to his inability to communicate and to his general disorganization. He gave the impression that he knew what he wanted to do and what he wanted to say, but that he was at a total loss to find his way out of the communication maze he was in, all of which increased his confusion and disorganization.

Not only was Dennis confused — he was confusing. His parents vacillated constantly in thinking that he might be deaf, suspecting that he might be mentally retarded, and wondering if he might be emotionally disturbed. This parental anxiety and disturbance also seemed to intensify Dennis's problem.

The psychologist who examined him indicated that Dennis had particular difficulty with tasks requiring the understanding or use of words and difficulty in perceiving similarities or differences in form, shape, and size of objects. Although Dennis tested in the retarded level on most tasks, and although his IQ score fell below normal, the psychologist believed that Dennis gave considerable evidence of "unavailable intelligence" and that he did not behave in ways typical of the mentally retarded child.

> 121   For further discussion of the responses of children with aphasia on mental tests and how they differ from mentally retarded children, read M. J. Berko, "Mental Evaluation of the Aphasic Child," *American Journal of Occupational Therapy*, V (1951), p. 6.

Dennis, like nearly all children suspected of having aphasia, was seen by a number of specialists, none of whom could claim him. The otologist's report stated that there was no anatomical or physiological reason for Dennis's lack of response to sound or speech, and a series of audiologic evaluations indicated that Dennis seemed to be "too deaf to be deaf." No overt neurologic signs were present, and the neurologist's report indicated that electroencephalographic studies were negative, with the exception of a "slight dysrhythmia."

Because no final conclusion could be reached concerning Dennis's severe delay in speech and language development, he was scheduled daily for three months of observational therapy designed to help him organize incoming information. This was done through matching, sorting, identification, and other similar activities.

> 122   For detailed discussions of methods used in the training and education of children with aphasia, read J. A. Hoffman, "Training of Children with Aphasic Understanding," *Nervous Child*, IX (1951), 85-88.

Following this three-month period, Dennis was re-examined, and at this time he was more tractable and he could be examined with less difficulty. His attention span had increased, his emotional outbursts had diminished, and, although he was still unable to use speech for communication, he seemed to understand some of the things which were said to him.

As indicated previously, Dennis is representative of only one type of aphasia in children. Other children may have a more severe receptive problem; some will have less difficulty understanding or comprehending words. Generally, the speech and language thera-

123   For another description of a child with aphasia, read G. W. Gens and
M. L. Bilbey, "Congenital Aphasia: A Case Report," *Journal of Speech and Hearing Disorders,* XVII (1952), 32-38.

pist should remember two key words: *confusion* and *organization.* The child is confused by verbal symbols; he needs help in organization. Therefore, the approach to the child with aphasia has three basic objectives:

First, the child with aphasia requires a special approach to his speech, language, and educational problem which is designed to provide meaningful experiences so that the child has an opportunity to associate verbal symbols (that is, words) with the appropriate objects, people, places, and things.

124   For a detailed description of one approach to this type of training,
read Hortense Barry, *The Young Aphasic Child: Evaluation and Training* (Washington, D. C.: The Volta Bureau, 1961).

Second, education of these children must be aimed at helping them organize incoming stimuli so that they can understand and comprehend incoming information for use in communication with others.

125   For specifics about an educational approach to these children, read
M. A. McGinnis, *Aphasic Children: Identification and Education by the Association Method* (Washington, D. C., The Volta Bureau, 1963).

And, third, these children must be introduced to a system whereby speech is no longer a rote articulation of sounds but, rather, a method of expressing ideas which are organized and meaningful.

126   Read H. R. Myklebust, *Auditory Disorders in Children* (New York:
Grune & Stratton, Inc., 1957).

DYSARTHRIA

A third type of problem associated with central nervous system impairment, and one which also results in delayed speech and language development, is the problem of *dysarthria*, a term used to describe motor involvement of the speech articulators.

127   Read W. G. Peacher, "Etiology and Differential Diagnosis of Dysarthria," *Journal of Speech and Hearing Disorders*, XV (1950), 252-65.

Gary was a dysarthric child referred to a speech and hearing clinic because his speech was unintelligible. He was a clumsy, awkward child who drooled profusely. Although he seemed to know what should be done with puzzles and form boards, he scored poorly on these tasks because of the time required for him to complete them. When he attempted to talk — which he did almost constantly — he was unable to manipulate his tongue or oral cavity, so that his speech was unintelligible. And he had other problems. For example, he was unable to chew meat or vegetables; therefore, most of the foods he preferred were soft ones, requiring no chewing and few swallowing movements. But even soft foods were difficult for him. For example, when he ate an ice cream cone, he moved the ice cream back and forth across his tongue, and he washed down any solid food with milk or water. Gary had to be taught how to move his tongue and lower jaw for speech articulation. This motor-kinesthetic approach entailed a long, repetitious series of procedures. It was necessary for him to learn to control the motor movements of his articulators, and this was accomplished through a step-by-step procedure.

128   Read M. Lefevre's article, "Language Problems of the Child with Cerebral Palsy," in N. E. Wood, *Language Development and Language Disorders* (Society for Research in Child Development, 1960).

Although central nervous system impairment was the causal factor for the delay in speech and language acquisition for all three of these children — Paul, Dennis, and Gary — the therapeutic approach to the problems of each was somewhat different. Paul required a broad-based educational approach — speech and language therapy was only one part. Dennis's problem required intensive language therapy, not only because of his inability to use symbols for speech, but also because it was expected that he might be found later to have a reading disorder. Gary's speech problem, on the other hand,

> 129   For information concerning early detection of reading disorders, read Katrina de Hirsch's test designed to discover potential reading difficulties at the six-year level, *American Journal of Orthopsychiatry*, LXXVII (1957), 409-13.

was more specific and related to motor dysfunction, for which speech therapy was his primary source of help.

> 130   For more information about dysarthria, read Muriel Morley, *The Development and Disorders of Speech in Childhood* (London: E. and S. Livingstone, 1957), which deals with the problems of children such as Gary.

MENTAL RETARDATION

There is general disagreement as to whether speech therapy can be beneficial to children who are mentally retarded. Some specialists insist that speech therapy for mentally retarded children, particularly those with IQ's below 70, is likely to be a waste of time. Others insist with equal confidence not only that children with IQ's as low as 50 benefit from speech therapy but that when they receive speech therapy routinely, their other educational problems become more easily managed. However, the problems of

> 131   For a more detailed discussion of the pros and cons of speech therapy for the mentally retarded, read J. Mathews' chapter, "Speech Problems of the Mentally Retarded," in L. E. Travis, *Handbook of Speech Pathology* (New York: Appleton-Century-Crofts, Inc., 1957).

mentally retarded children differ in terms of the factors which have caused the mental retardation. For example, consideration has been given to the differences between the language ability found in brain-

> 132   Read S. W. Bijou and H. Werner, "Language Analysis in Brain-Injured and Non-Brain-Injured Mentally Deficient Children," *Journal of Genetic Psychology*, LXVI (1945), 239-54. Additional information on this subject can be found in J. Weatherwax and E. P. Benoit, "Concrete and Abstract Thinking in Organic and Nonorganic Mentally Retarded Children," *American Journal of Mental Deficiency*, LXII (1957), 548-53.

injured mentally retarded children and the speech and language abilities of those children who are mentally retarded for reasons other than brain injury. Generally speaking, drill and repetition have formed the basic core of the therapeutic approach to speech stimulation for mentally retarded children, but also it is important that the speech and language therapist be aware of the differences between rote speech and communication. Hence, language therapy used with children with aphasia and other learning disorders has been found to be effective also with mentally retarded children, to some extent.

133   Read J. O. Smith, *Effects of a Group Language Development Program upon the Psycholinguistic Abilities of Educable Mental Retardates*, Peabody College Special Education Research Monograph, 1962, and "Speech Therapy with Mentally Retarded Children in Special Classes," by B. Schlanger, *Training School Bulletin*, L (1953), 179-86.

Children with mild to moderate retardation have been found to benefit from speech therapy, and specific attention to their speech and language development is conceded to be a necessary part of the total educational approach to their problem. For example, Billy was brought to a speech and hearing clinic for a speech and language examination because he was "slow" in speech development. He was small for his age and, perhaps because he was an attractive youngster, his mother had not considered the possibility that he was mentally retarded. Conferences with his mother revealed, however, not only that Billy was slow in speech development, but that he had been slow in other areas of development such as sitting and walking. Billy was a friendly child who tried through gestures and jargon to communicate, but the children in his neighborhood were not kind to him. This was due perhaps, to his inability to participate in group play. Usually he stood watching the other children running, jumping, and playing games but made no effort to join them on most occasions. When he did try to participate, the other children frequently shunned him and made fun of him because he could not talk. The more he tried to participate in neighborhood activities, the fewer were the children who paid attention to him.

When he was approximately five years of age, his mother took him for an examination by the school psychologist, a preparatory step for school entrance. She was told that Billy performed on most tests at a three-year, sometimes four-year, level, which placed him in the 70-85 range of intelligence scores. However, the psychologist pointed out that additional observations would be necessary before the degree of intellectual deficit could be pinpointed further. His

134   For an additional discussion of the evaluation of preschool children, read Elsa Hausermann, *Developmental Potential of Preschool Children; an Evaluation of Intellectual, Sensory, and Emotional Functioning* (New York: Grune & Stratton, Inc., 1958).

mother found this difficult to accept, because Billy was easily managed and generally cooperative. However, Billy did not remain the passive, smiling, accepting child that he once was. Because of his inability to communicate, and probably because of loneliness, since the other children would not include him in their play activities, he suddenly became extremely aggressive and difficult to manage. Other parents in the neighborhood would bring him home, complaining that he had attempted to bite or hit their children, and they demanded that Billy's mother keep him at home because they considered him a danger to the health and welfare of their own children. Disturbed, anxious, and unhappy about this course of events and no longer able to avoid or ignore the fact that Billy was not developing as other children of his age, his mother again consulted the school psychologist and finally accepted the fact that Billy was a mentally retarded child who needed help. One of the sources of help suggested was the speech and hearing clinic. After examination, Billy was scheduled for speech and language therapy with a small group of children, all of whom had some degree of mental retardation. Billy responded well in this speech-stimulation setting, and subsequent psychologic tasks substantiated some of the areas in which he had comparatively good competence. In spite of the fact that his mental retardation was a permanent problem, the speech and language therapist capitalized on his areas of strength, and he made gains in speech and language proportionate to his mental ability.

135   For more detailed information about procedures in speech therapy for mentally retarded children, read D. A. Weiss, "Speech in Retarded Children," *Nervous Child*, IX (1951), 21-30; and M. Bilbey, "A Rationale of Speech Therapy for Mentally Deficient Children," *Training School Bulletin*, XLVIII (1951), 236-39.

HEARING LOSS

Of all the causes of delayed speech and language development, perhaps the one which receives major attention from the speech and hearing therapist is the problem of hearing loss. Many fine texts have been devoted to the education of children with hearing impairment. Generally speaking, speech and language therapy,

136   For a comprehensive discussion of procedures used for the deaf and hard-of-hearing, read the two chapters by S. R. Silverman in L. E. Travis, ed., *Handbook of Speech Pathology* (New York: Appleton-Century-Crofts, Inc., 1957).

auditory training, and speech reading are integral parts of the education of the children with a severe hearing loss. The necessity for detecting the degree of hearing impairment is crucial to the types of therapeutic approaches used with these children.

137   For a discussion of a testing of hearing, read W. C. Hardy and J. E. Bordley, "Special Techniques in Testing the Hearing of Children," *Journal of Speech and Hearing Disorders*, XVI (June 1951), 122-31.

However, some children with delayed speech and language development may have a slight to moderate hearing loss which goes undetected because they learn to compensate for their hearing loss to some degree by using visual and tactual clues. Such was the case of Sharon, who appeared to be a bright youngster but a perplexed one. An unusually shy child, Sharon tended to stay close to her mother in all strange situations. In an effort to help her become better adjusted in social situations, her mother made arrangements for her to attend a nursery school. While at nursery school, Sharon either played quietly away from the other children or, if forced to participate in group activities, would usually cry and have to be taken to her mother for comfort. She played unusually well while alone and eventually, on a few occasions, was able to play cooperatively with one other child in activities such as building with blocks or coloring pictures. However, whenever speech was the focal point of the activity, she appeared lost and confused. The nursery school teacher suggested that Sharon have a physical examination. The pediatrician who examined her questioned her response to sound, and she was scheduled for a hearing examination. Audiologic examination revealed that Sharon had a mild to moderate hearing loss, and after being examined by an otologist, she was fitted with a hearing aid. Auditory training and speech therapy were recommended so that she could learn to make maximum use of her residual hearing. It was expected that speech would develop relatively rapidly at first, although it was also expected that discrimination between sounds which looked alike, or sounded alike, would continue to be difficult for her.

It is suspected that a large number of children may be delayed in speech and language development because of a slight to moderate hearing loss. Speech and hearing therapists must, therefore, be alert constantly to the possibility of these problems. Realistically, a slight hearing loss which is undetected may result in a much more exasperating problem than a severe hearing loss which has been recognized and diagnosed. Many children who have an undetected hearing loss may be thought to have aphasia, mental retardation, or emotional disturbance. To reduce the possibility of such diagnostic errors, children with delayed speech and language development should have a complete physical examination as well as audiologic and psychologic evaluations. Examinations of the child's mental abilities are of particular importance.

138   For more information about the nonverbal tests used for evaluating the mental abilities of children with hearing loss, read J. Snijders and N. Snijders, Non-Verbal Intelligence Tests for Deaf and Hearing Subjects (Groningen: J. B. Wolters, 1959).

EMOTIONAL DISTURBANCE

Emotional disturbance has been discussed previously, particularly severe disturbances such as symbiotic psychosis and autism. Yet, some children with comparatively mild emotional problems do not develop speech and language as expected. Many of these children require psychiatric care, and the speech therapist must be alert to certain behavioral patterns which support the need for psychiatric referral. Some of these clues are evident in the following description.

Everyone in the speech and hearing clinic knew that Steven was in the building five minutes after he had arrived. Concerned with the possibility that he might be separated from his mother, his anguished crying permeated every part of the clinic building. As he and his mother waited in the reception room, he alternated between pleading, clinging, whining, or crying, and actively attempting to pull his mother toward the door so that they could leave. He appeared to be extremely fearful of other people in the reception room, and he held onto his mother's arm with both hands. When he became convinced that he would not have to be separated from his mother, he quieted somewhat — enough so that the examiner could take both of them to the examination room. Once there, the examiner gave Steven some toys while both the examiner and the mother watched him while he attempted to play with them. But the toys had little meaning for Steven, and he manipulated the toy cars and trains in a disinterested manner, interrupting his activities by running frequently to his mother for attention. Once in a while he would say something to his mother, but he never spoke to the examiner. Whenever the examiner would say something to him, Steven's response usually was an echolalic one.

139   For more information about responses of emotionally disturbed children, read L. Kanner, *Child Psychiatry* (Springfield, Ill.: Charles C. Thomas, Publisher, 1948).

All of Steven's movements were quick and sure. If his mother so much as moved in her chair, he was quickly by her side, holding onto her or pulling her to the door of the examination room. Nothing could replace, even momentarily, his interest in being close to his mother. The examiner asked the mother to return to the clinic the next day, leaving Steven at home, so that they could discuss his problem without his being present. But Steven's mother said that she was unable to go anywhere without Steven — he even insisted on sleeping in her bed at night.

The mother discussed Steven's early development in the following way: he had been a very affectionate infant and he appeared to be developing normally until the birth of a second child when Steven was two years old. From that time on, Steven demanded almost uninterrupted attention from his mother. The second youngster was ill as an infant, requiring considerable care from the mother, and this seemed to accent Steven's problems. The mother believed that if Steven could learn to talk, this might help him "adjust." She reported that Steven had not been examined by a psychiatrist because she saw no reason for that type of examination. She also reported that no pediatrician saw either of her children routinely.

Considerable time was spent with the mother in pointing out the need for psychiatric examination prior to scheduling Steven for speech and language therapy. After several conferences, she agreed to have Steven examined by a psychiatrist, who supported the observations that Steven had an emotional problem requiring psychiatric care. The psychiatrist asked that the child be seen for speech and language therapy, preferably in a small stimulation group, while the psychiatric observations were being completed and prior to total recommendations and guidance for the parents.

> 140   For additional information along these dimensions, read J. T. Morrow, "A Psychiatrist Looks at the Nonverbal Child," *Exceptional Children,* XXV (1959), 347-51. Also read O. H. Mowrer, "The Autistic Theory of Speech Development and Some Clinical Applications," *Journal of Speech and Hearing Disorders,* XVII (1952), 263-68.

Speech therapy for children with emotional problems is more and more becoming recognized as a possible source of help for these children. Usually, the therapeutic setting is an extremely permissive one, and the children are encouraged to use speech only when they are ready for this form of communication. However, as is the case with some other causes of delayed speech and language development which have been discussed here, the speech therapist should have special training in the area of emotional disturbance so that the needs of these children will be understood and so that the stimulation of speech and language use will be compatible with some of the other types of therapy which these children might be receiving simultaneously.

IMMATURITY

A large number of the children who are brought to the attention of speech and hearing therapists have no apparent reason for their delayed speech and language development. Some of them have little or no need to use speech because their parents, siblings, relatives, and neighbors talk for them. Others are delayed temporarily in areas of development other than speech and language. Below are descriptions of two children whose delayed speech and language development is attributed to general immaturity.

Skip had little or no need to use speech for communication. He was the youngest child in his family, and he had five older brothers and sisters to talk for him. His mother, a large, overpowering woman, responded to Skip's every gesture and every whim. When he did attempt to communicate, he sounded like a slow motor boat as he vocalized "uh-uh-uh-uh" and pointed to the object he wanted.

Rather than attempt to use speech, he preferred to climb, no matter how high, to get an object rather than ask for it. His motor development was quite advanced, for these activities required considerable balance and motor skill. Although he stayed close to his mother, he did not hold onto her or attempt in any way to restrain her movements. To the contrary, his mother often held onto him. When asked about this overprotection, his mother explained that she feared something might happen to Skip, because he had no way to make his wants known. Skip's mother worried constantly about his health, and at the slightest sign of a sniffle or cough, Skip received considerable attention from his mother and older siblings. It was apparent that, at four years of age, he "ruled the roost." Yet, with all this attention, he did not appear to be a "spoiled" child but rather one who recognized that there was little need to use speech if others would speak for him or anticipate his needs.

Ellen was another example of an immature child. She had been a premature baby, and at five years of age her physical development was closer to that of a three-year-old. She, like Skip, had been cared for and coddled. She was thoroughly spoiled — in fact, she was a child tyrant. Intellectually she performed within normal limits, when tested, and there was no indication of a hearing loss. Ellen's parents reported that she had first begun to try to talk at three years. When she could not make herself understood, she would attempt to strike the person she was talking to or she would stamp her foot and kick until she got what she wanted. During the speech and language examination she could imitate most sounds in isolation. Pantomime and gestures were well developed, all of which her parents could understand readily.

Children like Skip and Ellen frequently benefit more from group activities than from individual therapy at least in the beginning. Most speech therapists are familiar with the so-called "speech-stimulation group" which usually consists of from six to eight children who are approximately the same age and who have approximately the same degree of delayed speech and language development. These groups usually are organized along the same educational dimensions as nursery schools, and speech therapists can benefit greatly by observing a normal nursery in action.

Speech and language development is, of course, the focal point of a speech-stimulation group, but perhaps the most important point which children learn in group situations is how to get along with other children their own age. Children learn from each other much more quickly than they learn from adults, and usually they insist on a "give and take" situation with their peers. A speech-stimulation group is, therefore, a good place for children like Skip and Ellen to learn that everyone is not going to talk for them. There they also learn that other children have the same kinds of difficulties as they are experiencing.

Speech-stimulation groups usually have activities which are play-oriented. The therapist may begin with group babbling, so that the children say sounds together: *ba-ba-ba-ba; da-da-da-da;* and so forth. Usually it is easier for children to make various combinations of sounds when they can do it with other children. Marching, finger painting, rhythm games, and cutting and pasting can be used for speech-stimulation purposes. Identifying sounds with pictures — cedure that speech therapists use effectively. Matching colors, then naming them; drawing pictures and coloring them — all activities which combine motor activities and speech sounds — have been found successful with these groups. Playing auditory games, where the child must identify the source of the sound produced by noise-makers while his back is turned, is another way to build up auditory memory patterns and sound-consciousness. In brief, any game, activity, or procedure which may be interesting to young children can be used effectively for speech-stimulation purposes.

141   For additional suggestions for ways to approach speech stimulation, read: M. C. Greene, *Learning to Talk* (New York: Harper & Row, Publishers, 1961), and C. Van Riper, *Speech Correction Principles and Methods,* 4th Ed. (Englewood Cliffs, N. J.: Prentice-Hall, Inc., 1963).

It is not possible to include here a detailed discussion of the various possible therapeutic techniques or approaches which might be effective with children with delayed speech. However, certain points have been emphasized here around which a speech and hearing therapist might formulate a basic philosophy about the therapeutic needs of children with delayed speech and language development.

In brief, therapy for children with delayed speech and language development must be tailored to the needs of each individual child *f-f-f* for the sound of a cat; *p-p-p* for the sound of a boat — is a pro- in accordance with the factors which have caused the delay in speech acquisition. It should be clear that there is no slick, isolated, failure-proof approach to all of these various problems. Speech and language therapists, therefore, must be knowledgeable in child development and have a keen awareness of the various causes of delayed speech and language development. They should be well-grounded in the various diagnostic procedures used to evaluate children with delayed speech and alert to the various differences in these children, if speech therapy is to be successful. In order to do this, it is necessary for the therapist to consider the goals and objectives for each child individually. The therapist should also be aware of the need for adequate facilities, equipment, and materials as an integral part of the therapeutic process, as well as for up-to-date records and progress reports which give a clear indication of both near- and long-term goals. Finally, the speech therapist must be aware of the need for a sound clinical relationship between therapist and parents, so that the child's parents can assume an instrumental role in reinforcing the therapeutic process at home. But, perhaps more than any other isolated factor, the speech and hearing therapist must recognize that all children with delayed speech and language development are alike in a few ways; that all children with specific disabilities which cause delayed speech and language development are alike in some ways; but that each child, regardless of cause or degree of involvement, remains a unique and separate individual whose problem must be approached in a unique and separate manner. ᘓᘓᘓ

bibliography

1. Albright, R. W. and J. B. Albright, "Application of Descriptive Linguistics to Child Language," *Journal of Speech and Hearing Research*, I (1958), 257-61.
2. Allerhand, M. E., "Psychological Assessment of the Non-Verbal Child," in N. E. Wood, ed., *Language Disorders in Children* (Society for Research in Child Development), XXV (1963), 49-57.
3. Anderson, R., "Report on the Development of a Communicative Evaluation Chart," *ASHA*, VI (1964), 81-83.
4. Bakwin, H., and R. Bakwin, *Clinical Management of Behavior Disorders in Children* (Philadelphia: W. B. Saunders Co., 1960).
5. Bangs, J. L., "Preschool Language Education for the Brain-Damaged Child," *The Volta Review*, LIX (1957), 17-19.
6. Bangs, T., "Evaluating Children with Language Delay," *Journal of Speech and Hearing Disorders*, XXVI (1961), 6-18.
7. Barger, W. C., "An Experimental Approach to Aphasic and to Non-Reading Children," *American Journal of Orthopsychiatry*, XXIII (1953), 158-70.
8. Barry, H., *The Young Aphasic Child: Evaluation and Training* (Washington, D. C.: The Volta Bureau, 1961).

9. Bayley, N., *The Development of Motor Abilities During the First Three Years* (Washington, D. C.: Society for Research in Child Development, 1935).

10. Benda, C., *Mongolism and Cretinism* (New York: Grune & Stratton, Inc., 1949).

11. Bender, L., *Psychopathology of Children with Organic Brain Disorders* (Springfield, Ill.: Charles C. Thomas, Publisher, 1956).

12. —— "Problems in Conceptualization and Communication in Children with Developmental Alexia," in P. H. Hoch, and J. Zubin, *Psychopathology of Communication* (New York: John Wiley & Sons, Inc., 1958).

13. Benton, A. L., "Aphasia in Children," *Education,* LXXIX (March 1959), 408-12.

14. Bergman, P., and S. Escalona, "Unusual Sensitivities in Very Young Children," *Psycho-analytic Study of the Child* (New York: International Universities Press), III (1949), 333-52.

15. Berko, F., and M. F. Palmer, "The Education of the Aphasic Child," *American Journal of Occupational Therapy,* VI (1962), 241-46.

16. Berko, M. J., "Mental Evaluation of the Aphasic Child," *American Journal of Occupational Therapy,* V (1951), 6.

17. Bilbey, M., "A Rationale of Speech Therapy for Mentally Deficient Children," *Training School Bulletin,* XLVIII (1951), 236-39.

18. Bijou, S. W., and H. Werner, "Language Analysis in Brain Injured and Non-Brain-Injured Mentally Deficient Children," *Journal of Genetic Psychology,* LXVI (1945), 239-54.

19. Bordley, J., and W. Hardy, "A Study of Objective Audiometry with the Use of a Psycho-Galvanic Response, *Annals of Otology, Rhinolaryngology, and Laryngology,* LVIII (1949), 751.

20. Bradley, C., "Organic Factors in the Psychopathology of Childhood," in P. H. Hoch, ed., *Psychopathology of Childhood* (New York: Grune & Stratton, Inc., 1955), 82-103.

21. —— "Characteristics and Management of Children with Behavior Problems Associated with Organic Brain Damage," *The Pediatric Clinics of North America,* I (November 1957), 1049-1060.

22. Caplan, G., ed., *Emotional Problems of Early Childhood* (New York: Basic Books, Inc., 1955).

23. Brown, R. *Words and Things* (Glencoe, Illinois Free Press, 1958).

24. Brown, S., ed., *The Concept of Congenital Aphasia from the Standpoint of Dynamic Differential Diagnosis,* a symposium published by the American Speech and Hearing Association, 1959.

25. Burke, M. F., "The Hyperkinetic Child," *Exceptional Children,* XXVII (September 1960), 18-26.

26. —— "The Effect of Brain Pathology on Learning," *Exceptional Children,* XXIV (1957), 169-72.

27. Carhart, R., "Speech Audiometry" *Acta Otolaryngology,* XLI (1953), 18.

28. Carrell, J. A., and J. L. Bangs, "Disorders of Speech Comprehension Associated with Idiopathic Language Retardation," *The Nervous Child, IX* (January 1951), 65-76.
29. Carroll, J., *The Study of Language: A Survey of Linguistics and Related Disciplines in America* (Cambridge: Harvard University Press, 1953).
30. Cattell, P., *The Measurement of Intelligence of Infants and Young Children* (New York: The Psychological Association, 1947).
31. Chreist, F., *Foreign Accent* (Englewood Cliffs, N. J.: Prentice-Hall, Inc., Foundations of Speech Pathology Series, 1964).
32. Clemmens, R. L., "Minimal Brain Damage in Children," *Children, VIII* (1962), 179-83.
33. Crabtree, M., *The Houston Test for Language Development* (Houston: Houston Press, 1963).
34. Cruickshank, W., and G. O. Johnson, eds., *Education of Exceptional Children and Youth* (Englewood Cliffs, N. J.: Prentice-Hall, Inc., 1958).
35. —— et al., *A Teaching Method for Brain-Injured and Hyperactive Children: A Demonstration Pilot Study* (Syracuse: Syracuse University Press, 1961).
36. Daley, W. T., ed., *Speech and Language Therapy with the Brain-Damaged Child* (Washington, D. C.: The Catholic University of America Press, 1962).
37. Darley, F., *Diagnosis and Appraisal of Communication Disorders* (Englewood Cliffs, N. J.: Prentice-Hall, Inc., Foundations of Speech Pathology Series, 1964).
38. Despert, J. L., *Emotional Problems in Children* (Utica: State Hospital Press, 1938).
39. Dimnet, E., *The Art of Thinking* (New York: Fawcett World Library, 1961).
40. Di Carlo, L., *The Deaf* (Englewood Cliffs, N. J.: Prentice-Hall, Inc., Foundations of Speech Pathology Series, 1964).
41. Doll, E. A., *Measurement of Social Competence* (St. Louis: Educational Publishers, Inc., 1953).
42. Doyle, P. J., "The Organic Hyperkinetic Syndrome," *The Journal of School Health, XXXII* (October 1962), 299-306.
43. Eisenberg, L., "Psychiatric Implications of Brain Damage in Children," *Psychiatric Quarterly, XXXI* (1957), 72.
44. Eisenson, J., "Aphasia and Dyslexia in Children," *Bulletin of the Orton Society, VIII* (1958), 3-8.
45. —— J. Ayer, and J. Irwin, "Language Development in the Child," *The Psychology of Communication* (New York: Appleton-Century-Crofts, Inc., 1963).
46. Ewing, A. W. G., *Aphasia in Children* (London: Oxford University Press, 1930).

47. Froeschels, E., *Dysarthric Speech* (Magnolia, Mass.: Expression Co., 1952).

48. Frostig, M., D. W. Lefever, and J. R. B. Whittlesey, "A Developmental Test of Visual Perception for Evaluating Normal and Neurologically Handicapped Children," *Perceptual and Motor Skills*, XII (1961), 383-94.

49. Gallagher, J., E. Benoit, and H. Boyd, "Measures of Intelligence in Brain-Injured Children," *Journal of Clinical Psychology*, XII (1956), 69-72.

50. ———— *A Comparison of Brain-Injured and Non-Brain-Injured Mentally Retarded Children on Several Psychological Variables*, Monographs of the Society for Research in Child Development (Yellow Springs, Ohio: The Antioch Press, 1957).

51. Gens, G. W., and M. L. Bibey, "Congenital Aphasia: A Case Report," *Journal of Speech and Hearing Disorders*, XVII (1952), 32-38

52. Gesell, A., and C. S. Amatruda, *Developmental Diagnosis* (New York: Paul B. Hoeber, Inc., 1957), 285-90.

53. Getman, G. N., and N. C. Kephart, *Advanced Tests of Visual Perception* (Loveland, Colorado: Childcare Co., 1963).

54. Goodenough, F. L., *Goodenough Draw-A-Man Intelligence Test* (New York: Psychological Corporation, 1957)

55. Greene, M. C., *Learning to Talk* (New York: Harper & Row, Publishers, 1961).

56. Hardy, W. C., and J. E. Bordley, "Special Techniques in Testing the Hearing of Children," *Journal of Speech and Hearing Disorders*, XVI (June, 1951), 122-31.

57. , ——— "Problems of Audition, Perception and Understanding," *The Volta Review*, LVIII (September 1956), 289-301.

58. Hardy, W. G., "An Analysis of Language Development in Children with Impaired Hearing," *Acta Otolaryngologica*, Supplementum 141 (1958), 51.

59. Haeussermann, E., *Developmental Potential of Preschool Children: An Evaluation of Intellectual, Sensory and Emotional Functioning* (New York: Grune & Stratton, Inc., 1958).

60. de Hirsch, K., "Gestalt Psychology as Applied to Language Disturbances," *Journal of Nervous and Mental Disease*, CXX (1954), 257-61.

61. ——— "Tests Designed to Discover Potential Reading Difficulties at the Six Year Level," *American Journal of Orthopsychiatry*, LXXVII (1957), 409-18.

62. Hoffman, J. A., "Training of Children with Aphasic Understanding," *The Nervous Child*, IX (1951), 85-88

63. Howard, R. W., "The Language Development of a Group of Triplets," *Journal of Genetic Psychology*, LXIX (1946), 181-88.

64. Howe, C. E., "A Comparison of Motor Skills of Mentally Retarded and Normal Children," *Exceptional Children*, XXV (1959), 352-54.

65. Johnson, W., F. Darley, and D. C. Spriestersbach, *Diagnostic Methods in Speech Pathology* (New York: Harper & Row, Publishers, 1963).
66. Kanner, L., "Early Infantile Autism," *Journal of Pediatrics*, XXV (1944), 211-17.
67. —— "Irrelevant and Metaphorical Language of Early Infantile Autism," *American Journal of Psychiatry*, CIII (1946), 242-46.
68. —— *Child Psychiatry* (Springfield, Ill.: Charles C. Thomas, Publisher, 1948).
69. Karlin, I. W., "Aphasias in Children," *American Journal of Diseases of Children*, LXXXVII (1954), 752-67.
70. Kastein, S., and E. P. Fowler, "Differential Diagnosis of Communication Disorders in Children Referred for Hearing Tests," *AMA Archives*, LX (1954), 468-77.
71. Kastenberg, J., "The History of an Autistic Child: Clinical Data and Interpretation," *Journal of Child Psychiatry*, III (1954), 5-52.
72. Kephart, N. C., *The Brain-Injured Child in the Classroom* (Chicago: National Society for Crippled Children and Adults, 1963).
73. Kirk, S. A., and G. O. Johnson, *Educating the Retarded Child* (Boston: Houghton Mifflin Company, 1951).
74. —— and J. McCarthy, "Illinois Test of Psycholinguistic Abilities — An Approach to Differential Diagnosis," *American Journal of Mental Deficiency*, LXVI (November 1961).
75. Kleffner, F., "Teaching Aphasic Children," *Education*, LXXIX (1959), 413-18.
76. Knobloch, H., and B. Passamanick, "Syndrome of Minimal Cerebral Damage in Infancy," *Journal of the American Medical Association*, CLXX (1959), 1384-7.
77. Laufer, M. W., "Hyperkinetic Behavior Syndrome in Children," *The Journal of Pediatrics*, L (April 1957), 463-74.
78. —— *et al.*, "The Hyperkinetic Impulse Disorder in Children's Behavior Problems," *Psychosomatic Medicine*, XIX (1957), 463-74.
79. Lerea, L., "Assessing Language Development," *Journal of Speech and Hearing Research*, I (1958), 75-85.
80. Lewis, M. M., *Infant Speech* (New York: Humanities Press, 1951).
81. Lewis, R. S., *The Other Child: The Brain-Injured Child*, Rev. Ed. (New York: Grune & Stratton, Inc., 1960).
82. Loomis, E. A., L. M. Hilgeman, and L. R. Meyer, "Childhood Psychosis: II. Play Patterns as Non-Verbal Indices of Ego Functions: A Preliminary Report," *American Journal of Orthopsychiatry*, XXVII (1957), 691-700.
83. —— "Autistic and Symbiotic Syndromes in Children," in N. E. Wood, *Language Disorders and Language Development*, Society for Research in Child Development, XXV (1960).
84. Luria, A. R., *Speech and the Development of Mental Processes* (London: Staples Press, 1959).

85. Mahler, M. S., "On Child Psychosis and Schizophrenia," *Psychoanalytic Study of the Child*, VII (New York: International Universities Press, 1952), 286-305.

86. Manteno, M. E., and J. Hazon, "Acquired Aphasia in Children," *Pediatric Americana*, III (1945), 188-92.

87. Marcus, R. E., D. L. Gibbs, and F. A. Gibbs, "Electroencephalography in the Diagnosis of Hearing Loss in the Very Young Child," *Disorders of the Nervous System*, X (1949), 170-73.

88. Masland, R. L., S. B. Sarason, and T. Gladwin, *Mental Subnormality: Biological, Psychological, and Cultural Factors* (New York: Basic Books, Inc., 1959).

89. Mathews, J., "Speech Problems of the Mentally Retarded," in L. E. Travis, ed., *Handbook of Speech Pathology* (New York: Appleton-Century-Crofts, Inc., 1957).

90. McCarthy, D., "Language Development in Children," in L. Carmichael, *Manual of Child Psychology* (New York: John Wiley & Sons, Inc., 1954).

91. ―――― "Language Disorders and Parent-Child Relationships," *Journal of Speech and Hearing Disorders*, IX (December 1954), 514.

92. McDonald, E., *Understand Those Feelings* (Pittsburgh: Stanwix House, Inc., 1962).

93. McGinnis, M. A., *Aphasic Children: Identification and Education by the Association Method* (Washington, D. C.: The Volta Bureau, 1963).

94. Meyers, R., and M. Meyers, "Adjustment Problems of the Aphasic Child," *The Crippled Child*, XXVIII (April 1951), 10.

95. Michal-Smith, H., and S. Kastein, *The Special Child* (New School for the Special Child, Inc., Bureau of Publications, 71 Columbia Street, Seattle 4, Washington, 1963).

96. Milisen, R., "Methods of Evaluation and Diagnosis of Speech Disorders," in L. E. Travis, ed., *Handbook of Speech Pathology* (New York: Appleton-Century-Crofts, Inc., 1957), 265-309.

97. Milman, J., "Organic Brain Disorder: Behavior Characteristics of Brain Damaged Children," *American Journal of Diseases of Children*, XCI (1956), 521-28.

98. Morley, M. E., *The Development and Disorders of Speech in Childhood* (London: E. and S. Livingstone, 1957).

99. ―――― D. Court, H. Miller, and R. F. Garside, "Delayed Speech and Developmental Aphasia," *British Medical Journal*, II (1955), 463-67.

100. Morrow, J. T., "A Psychiatrist Looks at the Nonverbal Child," *Exceptional Children*, XXV (1959), 347-51.

101. Mowrer, O. H., "The Autism Theory of Speech Development and Some Clinical Applications," *Journal of Speech and Hearing Disorders*, XVII (1952), 263-68.

102. ―――― "Hearing and Speaking: an Analysis of Language Learning," *Journal of Speech Disorders*, XXIII (1958), 143-52.

103. Myklebust, H. R., "Aphasia in Children," *Exceptional Children*, XIX (October 1952), 9-14.
104. —— *Auditory Disorders in Children* (New York: Grune & Stratton, Inc., 1954).
105. —— "Language Disorders in Children," *Exceptional Children*, XXII (1956), 163-66.
106. —— "Aphasia in Children — Language Development and Language Pathology," in L. E. Travis, ed., *Handbook of Speech Pathology* (New York: Appleton-Century-Crofts, Inc., 1957).
107. —— "Babbling and Echolalia in Language Theory," *Journal of Speech Disorders*, XXII (1957), 356.
108. —— and B. Boshes, "Psychoneurological Learning Disorders in Children," *Archives of Pediatrics*, VI (1960), 247-56.
109. —— *Training Aphasic Children* (Washington, D. C.: The Volta Bureau, Reprint No. 660, 1956).
110. Neilsen, J. M., *Agnosia, Apraxia, Aphasia: Their Value in Cerebral Localization* (New York: Hafner Publishing Co., Inc., 1962).
111. O'Leary, J., and Gitt, J., "Neurology in Office Practice," *General Practice*, VIII:4 (1954), 34-46.
112. O'Neill, J., *The Hard of Hearing* (Englewood Cliffs, N. J.: Prentice-Hall, Inc., Foundations of Speech Pathology Series, 1964).
113. Orton, S. T., *Reading, Writing and Speech Problems in Children* (New York: W. W. Norton & Company, Inc., 1937).
114. Osgood, C. E., and M. S. Miron, eds., *Approaches to the Study of Aphasia* (Urbana: University of Illinois Press, 1963).
115. Palmer, M. F., and F. Berko, "The Education of the Aphasic Child," *American Journal of Occupational Therapy*, VI (1952), 6, 6-7.
116. Peacher, W. G., "The Neurological Evaluation of Delayed Speech," *Journal of Speech and Hearing Disorders*, XIV (1949), 344-52.
117. —— "The Etiology and Differential Diagnosis of Dysarthria," *Journal of Speech and Hearing Disorders*, XV (1950), 252-65.
118. Pettit, C. W., "The Predictive Efficiency of a Battery of Articulatory Diagnostic Tests," *Speech Monographs*, XXIV (1957), 219-26.
119. Piaget, J., *The Origins of Intelligence in Children* (New York: International Universities Press, Inc., 1952).
120. Powers, M. H., "Functional Disorders of Articulation-Symptomatology and Etiology," in L. E. Travis, ed., *Handbook of Speech Pathology* (New York: Appleton-Century-Crofts, Inc., 1957).
121. *President's Panel on Mental Retardation: A Proposed Program for National Action to Combat Mental Retardation* (Washington, D. C.: U. S. Government Printing Office, 201, 1963).
122. Proceedings of the 1959 Annual Meeting of the Association for the Aid of Crippled Children, *The Child with Brain Damage* (New York: Association for the Aid of Crippled Children, 1961).
123. Rapin, I., "The Neurologist Looks at the Non-Verbal Child," *Exceptional Children*, XXVI (1959), 48-52.
124. Richardson, S. O., *Early Teaching for Children with Minor Central*

Nervous System Dysfunction (New York: United Cerebral Palsy Association, 1964).

125. Rooney, A. G., "An Aphasic Child in the School for the Deaf," *Volta Review,* XLVII (1945), 559-62.

126. Schiefelbusch, R. L., and H. V. Bair, "Language Behavior of Mentally Retarded Children," *Medical Times,* LXXXVIII (September 1960), 989-93.

127. Schlanger, B. B., "An Investigation of Retarded Brain-Damaged Children with Delayed Speech and Language," *Training School Bulletin,* LIII (May 1956), 64-74.

128. —— "Speech Therapy with Mentally Retarded Children in Special Classes," *Training School Bulletin,* L (1953), 179-86.

129. —— "Mentally Retarded and/or Aphasic," *Training School Bulletin* (1958), 62-65.

130. —— in Levin, *Voice and Speech Disorders: Medical Aspects* (Springfield, Ill.: Charles C. Thomas, Publisher, 1962).

131. Silverman, S. R., "Clinical and Educational Procedures for Hard of Hearing in Speech Pathology," in L. E. Travis, ed., *Handbook of Speech Pathology* (New York: Appleton-Century-Crofts, Inc., 1957).

132. Simon, C. T., "The Development of Speech," in L. E. Travis, ed., *Handbook of Speech Pathology* (New York: Appleton-Century-Crofts, Inc., 1957).

133. Smith, J., *Effects of a Group Language Development Program Upon the Psycholinguistic Abilities of Educable Mental Retardates* (Peabody College Special Education Research Monograph, 1962).

134. Snijders, J., and N. Snijders, *Non-Verbal Intelligence Tests for Deaf and Hearing Subjects* (Groningen: J. B. Wolters, 1959).

135. Solnitzky, O., "Disturbances of Language Formulation and Expression," *General Practice,* XIV (1956), 83-94.

136. Spitz R. A., "Hospitalism: An Inquiry Into the Genesis of Psychiatric Conditions in Early Childhood," *The Psychoanalytic Study of the Child,* I (New York: International Universities Press, 1945).

137. Stevens, S. S., and H. Davis, *Hearing* (New York: John Wiley & Sons, Inc., 1938).

138. Strauss, A. A., "The Education of the Brain-Injured Child," *American Journal of Mental Deficiency,* LVI (1951), 712-18.

139. —— and E. N. McCarus, "A Linguist Looks at Aphasia in Children," *Journal of Speech and Hearing Disorders,* XXIII (1958), 54-58.

140. —— and L. E. Lehtinen, *Psychopathology and Education of the Brain-Injured Child* (New York: Grune & Stratton, Inc., 1947).

141. —— and N. C. Kephart, *Psychopathology and Education of the Brain-Injured Child II: Progress in Theory and Clinic* (New York and London: Grune & Stratton, Inc., 1955).

142. Strother, C. R., *Neurologically Handicapped Child* (Chicago: National Society for Crippled Children and Adults, Inc., 1963).

143. Sugar, O., *Congenital Aphasia: An Anatomical and Physiological*

Approach," *Journal of Speech and Hearing Disorders,* XVII (1952), 301-304.

144. Templin, M., *Certain Language Skills in Children* (Minneapolis: University Minnesota Press, 1957).

145. Utley, J., *What's Its Name? A Guide to Speech and Hearing Development* (Urbana, Ill.: University of Illinois Press, 1950).

146. Van Riper, C., *Your Child's Speech Problems,* 4th Ed. (New York: Harper & Row, Publishers, 1961).

147. —— *Speech Correction Principles and Methods* (Englewood Cliffs, N. J.: Prentice-Hall, Inc., 1963).

148. —— *Teaching Your Child to Talk* (New York: Harper & Row, Publishers, 1950).

149. Weatherwax, J., and E. P. Benoit, "Concrete and Abstract Thinking in Organic and Non-Organic Mentally Retarded Children," *American Journal of Mental Deficiency,* LXII (1957), 548-53.

150. Weiss, D. A., "Speech in Retarded Children," *Nervous Child,* IX (1951), 21-30.

151. West, R., ed., *Childhood Aphasia: Proceedings of the Institute on Childhood Aphasia* (Gillick Printing, Inc., 1962).

152. Westlake, H., *A System for Developing Speech with Cerebral Palsied Children* (Chicago: National Society for Crippled Children and Adults, 1951).

153. Whatmough, J., *Language: A Modern Synthesis* (New York: Mentor Books, 1957).

154. Wood, N. E., "Causal Factors of Delayed Speech and Language Development," *American Journal of Mental Deficiency,* LXI (1957), 4-6.

155. —— "Language Disorders: An Education Problem," *Education,* LXXIX (March 1959), 399-403.

156. —— "The Child with Aphasia," *The Journal-Lancet,* LXXIX (July 1959), 315-17.

157. —— *Language Disorders in Children* (Chicago: National Society for Crippled Children and Adults, 1959).

158. —— *Language Development and Language Disorders,* Society for Research in Child Development (April 1960).

159. —— "Language Disorders: Major Barriers to Communication," *School Life,* VI (1961), 43.

160. —— "Educational Evaluation of School Aged Children with Language Disorders," in W. Dayley, ed., *Speech and Language Therapy with the Brain-Damaged Child* (Washington, D. C.: The Catholic University Press, 1962).

161. —— "Decision Making: Childhood Aphasia," *ASHA,* V (April 1963), 571-75.

162. Yates, A. J., "Disorders of Speech, Brain Damage and Learning Theory," *Education,* LXX (1959), 444-47.

163. Young, C., and McConnell, F., "Retardation of Vocabulary Development in Hard of Hearing Children," *Exceptional Children,* XXIII (1957), 368-70.

index

index